DO WE REALLY NEED BOTOX?

A Handbook Of Anti-Aging

A Gift to Hagar's Foundation for Single Mothers

Volume 1.0

SOFIA DIN, MD

Disclaimer:

The information in this book is of a general nature and is intended to help you understand issues around health, anti-aging, aesthetic medicine, and nutrition; it is not a substitute for professional advice. The publisher and author accept no liability for damages arising from the information in this book. Please always consult your doctor and/or a health professional for advice specific to your individual health requirements.

CONTENTS

Acknowledgements   v

Dedication cum Prologue
vii

Introduction: What is Anti-Aging, and Why Does it Matter?
1

1   Body Dysmorphia—How to Learn to Walk with Your Demons
27

2   Do we Really Need Botox?
45

3   Filters, Fillers, and Facelifts. Stop Waiting for Easier Solutions.
65

4   Allergan, I love you. Allergan, I hate you.
79

5   Food for Thought
85

6   Weight Loss Without Fat Shaming
117

7   Skin-Tightening Devices
139

8   Find Your Missing Pieces: Find Your Tribe and Unfollow the Joneses
143

ACKNOWLEDGEMENTS

Writing this book while working full-time often felt like childbirth. I couldn't have done it alone. It took a town to get the book to the shape it has now that you hold it in your hands, looking whole without obvious deformities. I am ever so grateful to so many people, more than I could possibly acknowledge here, who came together to help me deliver my first book. Many of them are my clients who saw me super busy, super-focused, often rushing, sometimes frantically to keep my businesses and my affairs running smoothly. They offered to help. They read the manuscript carefully and being familiar with my work and philosophy, they helped give shape to the work. And then some people really stepped in when they saw me struggling to finish this project for the non-profit foundation.

So my special thanks go to David Peritz for co-authoring the chapters on "Food" and "Missing Pieces" with me. I am eternally grateful to Muisi Krosi, Tom Augst, Michael Perez, and Bethany Brown for helping me with final editing. I must thank my amazingly wonderful staff who helped me in innumerable ways. Last but not the least I am grateful to my daughter Lyla, who told me to be completely true to myself as to my readers, and write the way she writes in her still unpublished, personal journals.

DEDICATION CUM PROLOGUE:
To Hagar, the Original Single Mother and the Eternal Immigrant

Who was Hagar? There are various religious stories about her origin, but everyone agrees that she was an Egyptian and that she was given to the Prophet Abraham to serve as the handmaiden of his wife, Sarah. Hagar was very beautiful and also quite resourceful. Muslims believe that she was married to the Prophet Abraham to be the surrogate to bear him a son named Ishmael. His first wife, Sarah was anxious about her own aging, and feared that the prophecy that she will give Abraham a son might not come to pass. This is why she arranged to involve Hagar. Yet, despite her worrying, Sarah did in fact become pregnant some years later, giving birth to a son named Isaac. Both women started disliking each other, and Sarah ultimately asked Abraham to get rid of Hagar. (This is not the first time two strong women fought over a man, where one of them won and the other one had to move on.)

So Abraham abandoned Hagar and their son, Ishmael, in the desert with some food and water, and nothing else. Their meager supplies didn't last long, and Hagar desperately searched for water, becoming frantic as fear for her son's life escalated. That is when a spring miraculously appeared. This spring had flowed there all along, but in her heightened state of anxiety, Hagar was unable to see it. The water helped her realize that her son would be safe. She was able to calm herself down. She became reconciled to God's will and accepted that Abraham would never return. Hagar and Ishmael eventually settled down to a new life. Ultimately, Ishmael married a very beautiful girl.

Hagar is recognized in all three Abrahamic religions—Judaism, Christianity, and Islam. Arabs call her Hajjara, and consider the spring she found to be holy. During Hajj, the annual pilgrimage to Mecca that Muslims are required to make at least once in their lifetime, believers retrace Hagar's search for water by rushing seven times between the hills of Safa and Marwa. This ritual is said to honor Hagar, commemorating her journey, her thirst and suffering. Tradition reports that the Prophet Muhammed himself instructed followers to observe this ritual during their pilgrimage, as it was revealed to him that he himself was a direct descendant of Hagar's.

The soul of Hagar's story resonates with my own life's journey. Although I no longer consider myself a single mother since I am now in a healthy & a mutually nurturing relationship. But pretty much throughout my married life I felt completely alone and left to fend for myself and my daughter, so I came to empathize with the burdens, vulnerability and angst of single mothers. As a doctor I made enough money to be able to throw it at some of my problems, but even though money didn't fix all my problems, it did help make life somewhat comfortable, and then I met so many women who couldn't afford to do the same. This lead me to start a Foundation for Single mothers and to write a book to create revenue for workshops. The proceeds of this book will go entirely to Hagar's Foundation, which will provide a source of support and guidance to single mothers. And just as Hagar was a believer in the divine light and mercy of the Almighty, I will seek to follow her light.

Having been blessed with professional success, while also arriving at a place of personal happiness and fulfillment, I plan to eventually retire as a social entrepreneur. During my years of practice, I have found that what is profitable may not be healthy, and vice versa. As a solo practitioner, I cannot change the healthcare system, but I can work to change the focus of my own practice and follow a not-for-profit model. I will be reworking important aspects of my anti-aging practice to make its services more readily available and useful to single mothers.

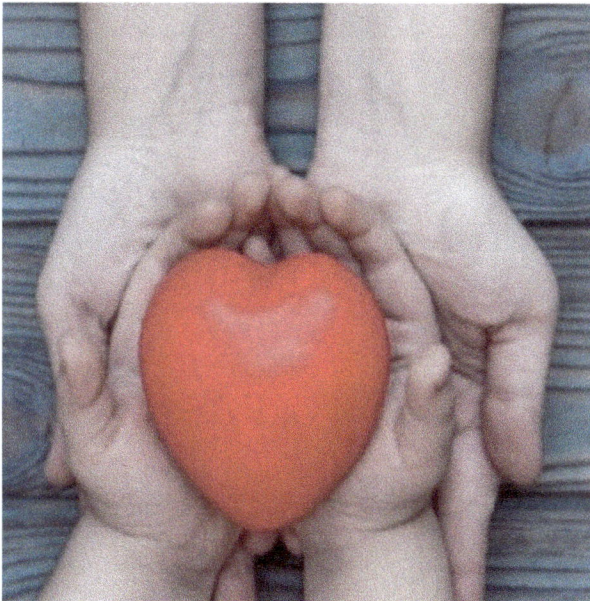

In this phase of my career, as I continue to serve all people, I will especially dedicate myself to supporting single mothers so that they can live their lives with purpose, vitality, and overall wellness. I extend my support by continuing to employ single mothers at my medical practices. I recognize they have unique struggles and needs as they enter the workforce and try to advance professionally. To help address these barriers, one of the first programs to be implemented at Hagar's Foundation is a job interview preparation package. Résumé writing, interview preparation, and coaching services are provided. Additionally, salon services, such as hair styling and makeup, can be provided in preparation for the interview. We even assist with fresh, dry-cleaned clothes, if needed. We charge one-third the cost of market value of providing these services and, in certain deserving cases, we ask them to help someone else later on by paying it forward. Other programs at Hagar's Foundation include life coaching, health and wellness coaching, financial literacy, and meditation and emotional intelligence workshops. These are areas of support that women need in general, but especially women in complex societies, who have to fend for themselves financially. I hope you will decide to purchase this book because you are curious about the approach it offers: rethinking the relationship between medicine, anti-aging, and well-being; but you can also feel good knowing that the proceeds go to making services like these available to those who need them but cannot otherwise afford them.

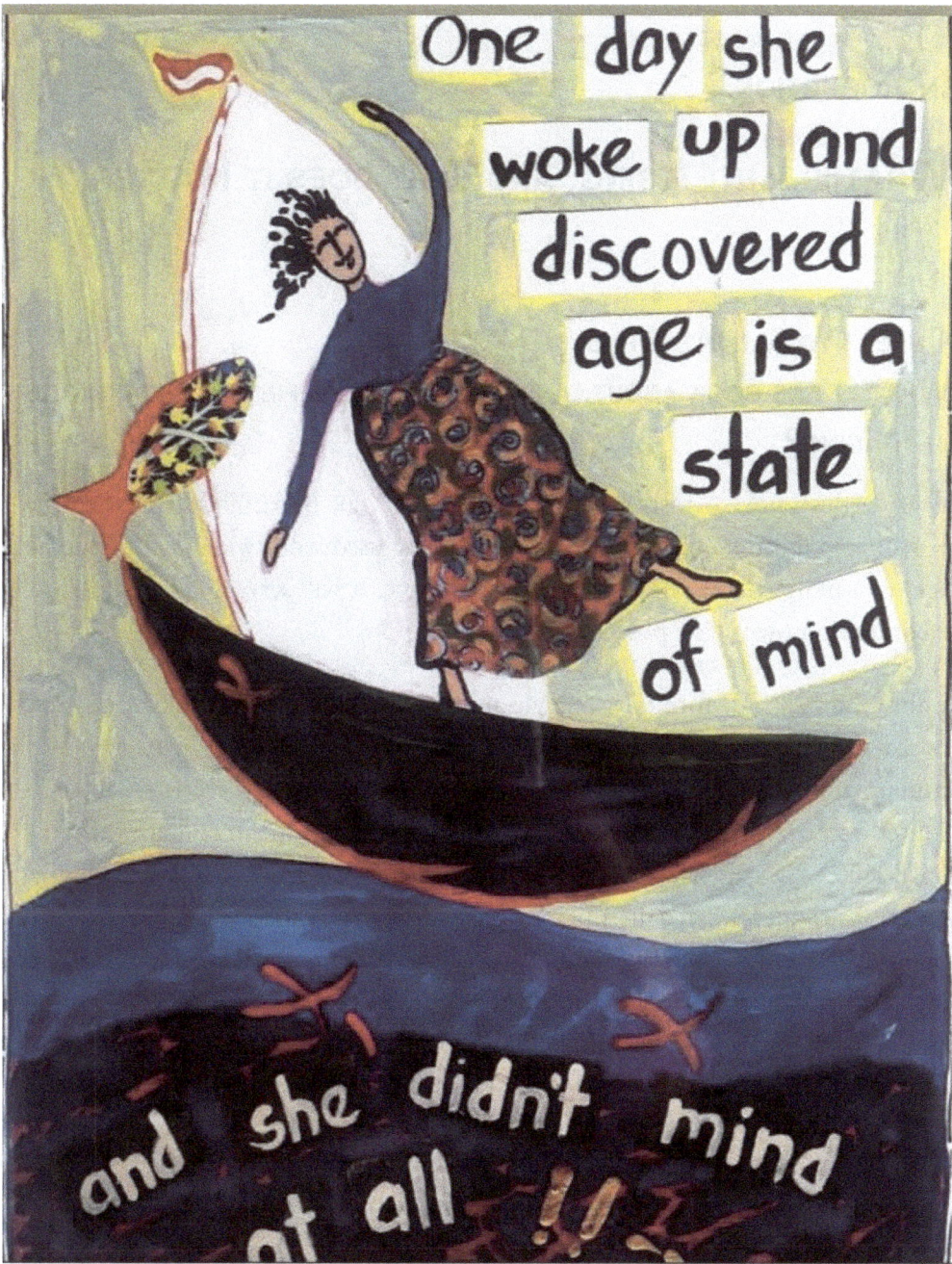

One day she woke up and discovered age is a state of mind

and she didn't mind at all!!!

9

WHAT IS ANTI-AGING, AND WHY DOES IT MATTER?

CHEERS TO ALL MY WHYS:
WHAT IS THIS BOOK ABOUT, AND WHY AM I QUALIFIED TO SPEAK ABOUT ANTI-AGING?

I wrote this book to instruct as well as amuse you, hopefully simultaneously. In it, I explain and illustrate procedures currently being used worldwide in efforts to help people age with more energy, vitality, beauty, and grace. It will serve as a handbook to help you navigate your own aging process.

I am a 48-year-old, formerly a single mother of a now 20-year-old young lady. I am a board-certified family medicine doctor who has been directly managing the health of patients over the past 15 years in New York; I also served as a Geriatrician and a Medical Director of a Nursing Home for 6 years. This brought me in contact with patients not only acutely sick in hospitals, while others were seen in my clinics, or as they became functionally incarcerated in nursing homes. I have experienced healthcare systems at opposite extremes—in Pakistan, my country of origin, where I originally trained in medicine and surgery, and in the United States, where I re-established myself as a doctor and completed residency training again before establishing my practices. I now own and manage a medical practice as well as an anti-aging/wellness center.

I have no Yale or Harvard degrees to boast of, since I am an immigrant from Pakistan. However, I have worked very diligently and consistently over the years to gain mastery in the fields of primary care, geriatrics, aesthetics, and anti-aging, while honing my medical skills and techniques. I know some will suspect that a doctor writing a book like this one is engaged in self-promotion, advertising their practice to drum up more business, and so they may not take it seriously for the anti-aging philosophy and medical advice it contains. My practice is already quite busy and has a great retention rate in a very competitive market, due to the high quality of our services and products. This book is not an advertising tool for me or even for Hagar's Foundation (which is a non-profit resource center for single mothers). It contains parts of my own life's journey, and imparts some of the inside knowledge and skills I gained as I helped and cared for other human beings as a doctor, and it is my intention to try to change the way medical care is currently understood, provided, and funded beyond the confines of my own practices.

My approach to medicine, especially in the areas of aesthetics and anti-aging, grows directly out of my experiences as a woman and as a doctor. As a woman, growing up in Pakistan wasn't easy. Although blessed with an educated family that allowed me to go to school, I suffered from low self-esteem and mild depression much of my life. This made me very introverted. I also suffered from psoriasis, an autoimmune skin disorder that leads to scaly patches that make you look as if your skin is disintegrating. Imagine a young adult with sloughing skin all over her body. It was much worse than facial acne. (I also suffered from that every now and then.) Battling a chronic skin disorder, especially when young, is an awful experience. One never gets better. No topicals or pills work, and every treatment has a list of side effects galore that can make you sick, just from reading it. At least that was my reaction. My brain and my immune system played havoc with me as I struggled through high school, college, and medical school.

I've always had a strong spirit, but this is not always an asset for a woman in certain cultures and contexts. So even though I am a firm believer in marriage, and upholding our sacred vows, my list of accomplishments includes two failed arranged marriages. As a young and self-conscious woman, I had low self-esteem, so I never really looked for a boyfriend. The boys I liked didn't really like me all that much, and I didn't like the ones I ended up marrying. For me, arranging to marry the second husband felt like taking a second job: signing the contract, getting housing, health insurance, and even the possibility of having a child that I can call my own. Instead of being exciting, I found my marital career totally toxic and negative. My environment was very unpredictable, and could turn violent, since he had anger management issues. Testosterone in men is not always a blessing.

But it wasn't altogether bad; coming to America to marry my second husband was also a second chance at life. Americans celebrate Independence Day on July 4, but I celebrate it again on October 10—the day I got on the plane and came to New York. No matter how difficult my personal life got in New York, it was always better than where I had come from, and it ultimately allowed me to make the life I now love. After the birth of my daughter, my psoriasis pretty much went away; motherhood and its hormones came like a blessing for my body. Eventually, after 13 years, I divorced my second husband. We became much more friendly with each other after our divorce. The loss of marriage, perhaps, broke him down a bit, and he became a nicer person to me. My daughter found it much more pleasant when we were divorced and not taking each other for granted or openly hostile. Unfortunately, he suddenly passed away in 2014, leaving my then 15-year-old daughter in a spiral of grief. But my divorce helped me with my depression and self-doubt. I started realizing that good things start happening when you protect yourself from toxic circumstances, start viewing yourself through your own eyes instead of others, and create spaces of love, support, and success for yourself. It was slow and intense work and thankfully, I was able to transfer this awareness to my daughter as well, who went through various stages of complicated grief during her life-altering teenage years and still managed to be emotionally strong enough to land on her feet and start flourishing.

I always knew that I was going to be a doctor, and I was driven from a young age. When I was only four years old, I asked my mom for a syringe and a stethoscope so I could fix my little sister. My parents were not interested in getting me any toys. They were the original authors of Desi Austerity 101. (*Desi* derives from the Hindi word for "country" and is used to refer to people of Indian and Pakistani descent.) I waited for six years, before I finally got my first stethoscope and doctor toy set when I was 11 years old. In the subsequent years, I also managed to somehow become a doctor in Pakistan despite suffering from mild depression and low self-esteem due to my skin condition and a broken first marriage.

During my very short-lived (year-long) first marriage, I heard someone mention how they got married to someone in America, got a green card, and moved there. A light bulb lit up in my head. Could I do that, too? Move to the Land of the Free and the Brave? Will Lady Liberty accept the wretched waste that my existence had been so far? After my first divorce, as I struggled to finish medical school in Pakistan, my mom told me about a proposal by a 37-year-old young and charming Kashmiri New Yorker. He was also a Wharton School of Business graduate and worked as an accountant. I readily said yes. I was also going to be his second wife. He had a failed, short-lived previous marriage from which he had two beautiful kids, a boy and a girl, who lived with his ex-wife. So I moved to America for this arranged and, as it turned out, mainly unhappy marriage. I was blessed with a girl-child, whom I wanted to raise in America, so that she might have a better cultural environment than my country of birth. I decided that my best option was to change my job from that of a housewife to a doctor again. This would help me to become financially independent of my second husband, who was quite temperamental and emotionally unstable. Practicing medicine again was my ticket to freedom and happiness.

To practice medicine in America, there were rules. You needed to prove your "rite of passage" by taking a series of extremely difficult exams. So after going through seven years of medical school, I had to re-take all examinations in the U.S. before I could even apply to train in a residency program. Residency programs are designed as a way to monitor and train new doctors under supervision before they are allowed into the United States healthcare system. This meant taking the U.S. Medical Licensing Exams and completing a residency training, and it was not at all easy. The first step was especially a challenge for me because the USMLEs are not only inherently difficult, but they are also the product of a totally different system of education and test-taking than I was used to back in Pakistan. Plus, I had a very mild case of dyslexia since I was a child. Initially, I attributed this to being multilingual, but as I got older, I became aware of how slow my brain processed written words, and it took me literally twice as long to read what others could read fairly quickly. Despite this, through long and hard work, I was able to compensate for my dyslexia, and I completed medical school.

The Pakistani system of education is predominantly British, and it places more emphasis on thought building, essay writing, and getting your message across, etc. But Americans were not about that life. This was especially true in New York, where everything was simply faster. No one took the time to breathe deeply and absorb the magnificence that surrounded them. Even the testing process encouraged rapid memorization and regurgitation, not practical skill or reflection. There are three USMLEs and each is nine hours long. Doctors answer 50 questions in 60 minutes for nine hours with very few breaks for food. I mean, what's up with all the multiple choice questions that you have to answer within a minute? Robots and computers can do it much better than humans. But I would wonder if robots could really connect with a human being and solve their problems with empathy, love, and grace like a fellow human could? *Anyway, long story short, overcoming my partial dyslexia to re-establish myself as a doctor in America was nothing less than learning mental acrobatics all over again, only this time while being a new wife and a new mother in a new country.*

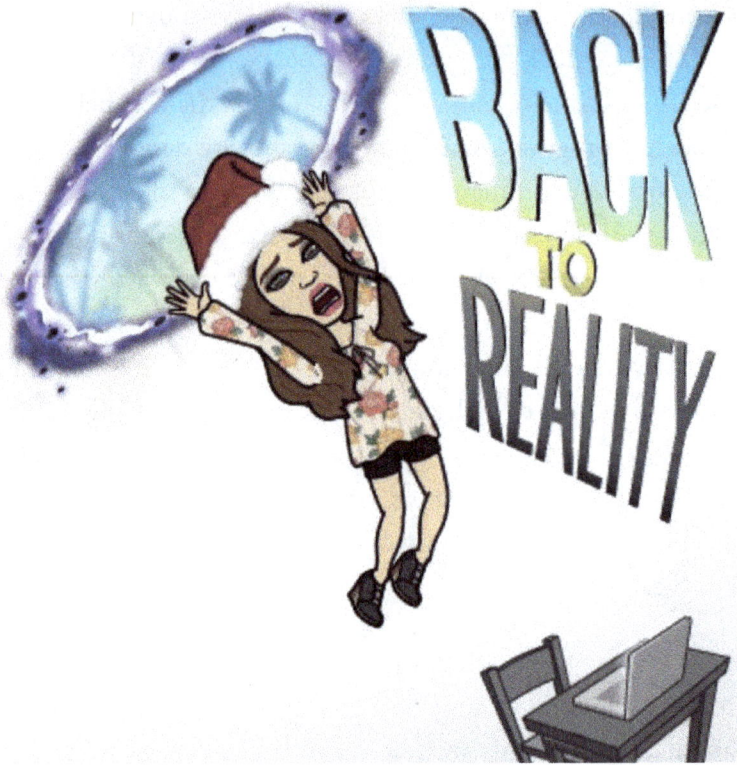

After completing my recertification, I managed to find a residency training program in family medicine close to my house. This meant I could still manage to look after my daughter, who was only three years old at the time. Landing a residency program 20 minutes away from my home was such a blessing. I knew my then-husband would never allow me to move to another state and I would have to battle for the safety of my child. By the way, finding residency while competing with American medical graduates is also not easy. These are young, energetic, and well-trained individuals who have bought their rites of passage into healthcare by paying their dues at big American medical institutions. I still remember Dr. Joseph Halbach, who selected me into the residency program and gave me a chance to free myself from the economic bondage of my second husband. After completing residency, I decided to open my own practice. I did not want to take up any jobs working for someone else. I had already tried out two toxic marital careers, and serving another person or organization was not a choice for me, not even to gain experience.

things I needed to hear 5 years ago

by chibird

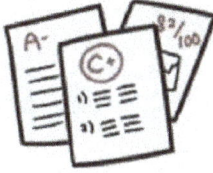

you won't even
remember these grades

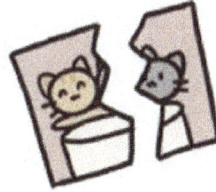

not every friend
is forever

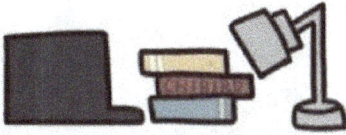

your hard work
does pay off

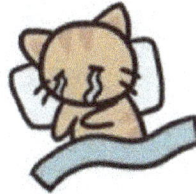

it turns out okay,
I promise.

Since my husband did not support my life's ambitions on an emotional or financial level, I needed to find other sources of support. I was able to borrow money from my girlfriend, Sophia, (half her paycheck for several months) to start my own medical practice. I worked consecutive shifts at my own practice and as a hospitalist to pay for office overhead. All that work allowed me to gain experience and grow my business quickly. At the same time, I was invited to become the medical director of a nursing home and medical rehab center. This was a large facility that cared for the elderly and also provided post-operative and protracted illness care. I served an aging and sick population for almost six years. My practice had its own wound care doctor, nurse practitioner, and some really experienced doctors to advise me as we began managing geriatric health. I also tended to patients at St John's Riverside Hospital close to my office in Yonkers. First, I served as an attending physician, then as faculty, and finally on their board. In all of these contexts, I managed acutely sick patients alongside trusted colleagues.

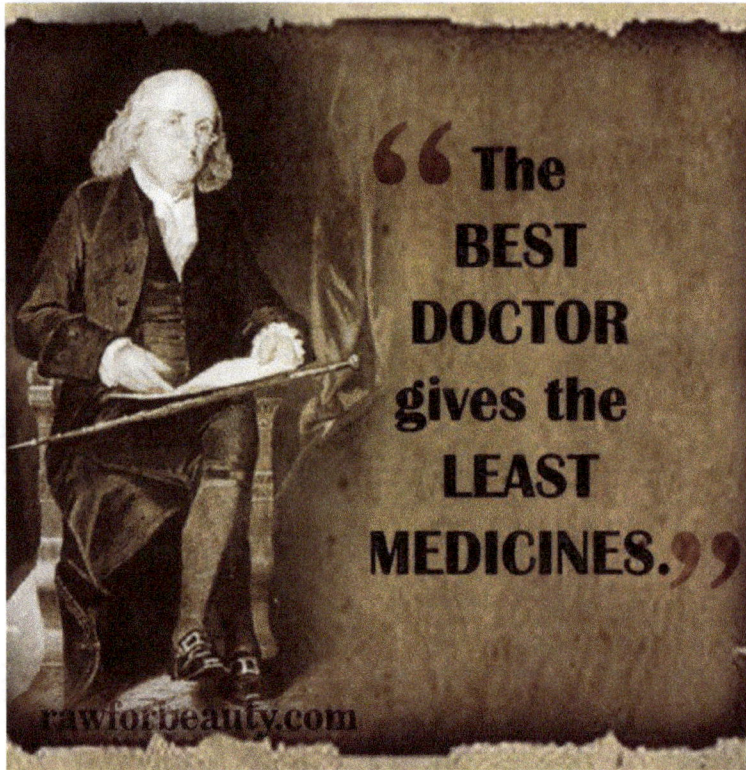

From these diverse and extensive experiences, I learned one overarching lesson: Healthcare in the United States operates mainly as sickness management. Once you get sick, insurance companies start paying for medications, tests, admissions, and doctors. No one is bothered about your wellness or anti-aging or overall well-being. There were other lessons life had taught me up to this point, perhaps most importantly the relationship between the way others see you and the way you see yourself, and its impact on your self-esteem. I learned about the need to have control and agency over central circumstances of my life. These combined realizations led me first to start a second practice with an exclusive focus on well-being, anti-aging, and aesthetics (Juvanni Med Spa and Anti-Aging Center). As part of this work, I undertook a systematic study of types of medical care that are mainly neglected and certainly not covered within the American healthcare system. And, to jump briefly ahead to the present, eventually I founded Hagar's Foundation for Single Mothers so that at least some of those who cannot afford to pay for this kind of care out of pocket are not denied access to it.

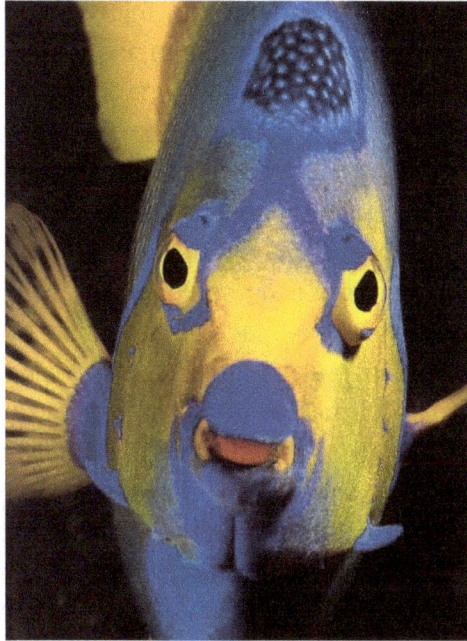

Many family members questioned me about sharing my story with the world as I invoked their support for my cause. Why do you have to tell people about your past? I had heard Hasan Minhaj's (a very famous and popular comedy show host of Indian descent) talking about his parents' reaction to some personal event on an episode: "log kiya kahein ge?" or "What will people say?" My mom would say exactly the same thing, and I would tell my mom: How can I convince people to follow my advice if they don't know who I am or why I am saying what I am saying? My credibility has to be established by my work and, also, my narrative about my life and work. It is only then that I can gain their trust for the advice I offer and seek their support in my cause.

So what is my cause? *As a doctor, I believe in disease-free aging for everyone, and this is the focus of this book. I also wish to spread awareness about aging. I believe that Aging is a disease in itself which leads to several signs and symptoms which manifest as diseases. From the moment of our birth our cells and bodies begin to age. After 40 this process accelerates a bit, and after 65 it accelerates even faster. When our cells age, they grow weaker, and like an old computer disc that can't pay the music because of all the scratches on it, our chromosomes and DNA gets unraveled and is unable to produce the chemicals and proteins that we need to function in a healthy way. When our bodies are young, there is continuous production of new cells that replace the old ones, but as we get older, and the majority of our cells are now old, we tend to decline faster and become weak.* There is something wrong with the way we age - and the way the healthcare system deals with aging. On one hand, doctors get paid once their patients already have a disease, injury or ailment; the entire healthcare system is built on the treatment of poor health, instead of prevention, and as a result, important emerging preventative measures are not covered by insurance but instead treated as luxury services. This systematic flaw in ideas about health and healthcare impacts how we age at a moment when humans are living longer and longer. Our brain doesn't like to have a discrepancy in its perception of reality and reality itself. When people internalize a conception of themselves as old or aged due to the unconscious self-image generated by seeing lines, wrinkles, and saggy skin in the mirror, many start manifesting a cascade of events biologically that lead to continued aging. We can actually age ourselves faster by perceiving ourselves as old in the first place. *My clinical practice is built on the idea that taking anti-aging measures can prevent the effects of aging on the entire body.* I believe other health practitioners should join me in treating aging itself as a disease, and we should work to figure out what causes aging in order to systematically tackle its signs and symptoms by using the healthcare system to its fullest capacity, and by addressing how we perceive our own aging bodies. If we consider aging a disease, then anti-aging treatments would be better supported by the healthcare system instead of being characterized as elective or optional, making them more accessible to everyone. It's time that we accept aging as the disease it is, so we can finally start treating it like one.

And in my foundation (which the proceeds of this book support), I am focused on helping single mothers who need to live with energy, health, wellness, vitality, and success—for their own sake as well as that of their children. I consider single mothers to be especially vulnerable to poor mental and physical health outcomes.. Therefore, the mission of Hagar's Foundation is devoted to the welfare of single mothers everywhere. Our future programs will be designed to help single mothers around the world, and currently we are focusing on programs to help single moms get good jobs.

But first let's figure out what *anti-aging* really is.

The dictionary says that "it's a product or a technique that is designed to prevent the appearance of getting old."[1] **Why is preventing the *appearance* of getting old important?** In my opinion, it is very important for us to make ourselves look youthful because our brains work in a very strange way. Philosophy, psychology, and medicine agree on the central importance of how you think of yourself—your self-conception—to how you feel, what you do, and how you react in different situations, etc. If your brain begins to internalize an old or aging image of yourself, your self-conception may shift

---

[1] For a more extensive discussion of anti-aging, see: David A. Sinclair, *Lifespan: Why We Age——and Why We Don't Have To,* (NP: Atria Books, September 10, 2019).

subconsciously in the direction of what you think old people are like. This can cause distress and even start a cascade of signs and symptoms that will manifest as diseases of old age like osteoporosis, heart disease, cognitive decline and dementia. It doesn't help that our culture idolizes youth and presents us with few images of older adults as vital and attractive.

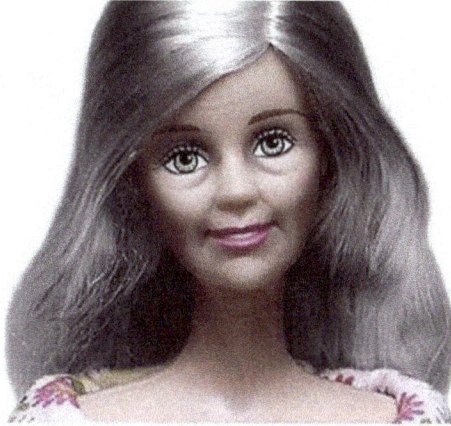

drnaomi1
Sydney Australlia

BARBIE AGE 42. DIDN'T DO ANYTHING TO HER SKIN WHEN SHE WAS YOUNGER BECAUSE SHE HAD *GOOD SKIN ALREADY*.

As a result of a shift in your implicit self-conception, you can start feeling tired and perhaps even experience greater susceptibility to chronic and potentially life-threatening illnesses and diseases. Despite being ill, the modern healthcare system won't allow you to die that fast, as there are antibiotics, chemotherapy, painkillers, sleeping pills, blood thinners, anti-cholesterol medications, and mind-numbing agents like anti-anxiety meds. Additionally, there are some very cool technologies that will surely keep you alive, at least 25 to 35 years longer than your brain wants you to live. *I tell my patients and clients that either you will spend money on your health or on your sickness.* But, once you're sick, you will spend a lot of money keeping yourself alive irrespective of the quality of life that results.[2]

---

[2] On this theme, see the wonderful work of Atul Gawande, *Being Mortal: Medicine and What Matters in the End*, (London: Picador, 2015).

But since maintaining the appearance of our skin and other aspects of physical vitality are not considered medical concerns, very little emphasis is placed on the upkeep of our facial skin, etc. as we age. In my opinion, that's a flawed stance.

How our brains view ourselves and how others view us can translate into the rapid progression of aging. As the field of neuroscience is developing, our understanding of mirror neurons is also advancing. My hypothesis, developed in chapters below, is that mirror neurons may play an important part in an *aging syndrome*, where symptoms associated with aging, such as fatigue, chronic aches and pains, sleep disorders, and perhaps even greater susceptibility to chronic illness and disease, start manifesting as the brain internalizes an understanding of yourself as aged and infirm based on the way it processes and reacts to your aging face and other seemingly superficial signs of aging.

Maslow's Hierarchy of Needs

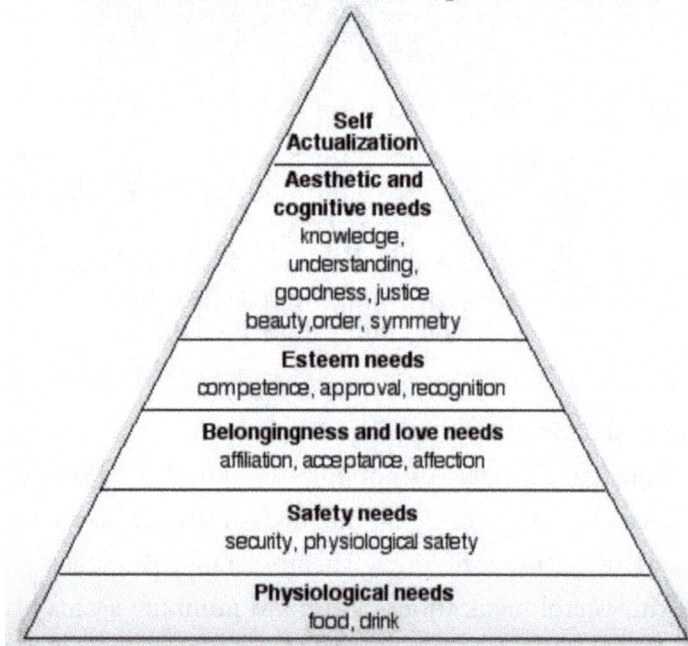

Self Actualization

Aesthetic and cognitive needs
knowledge, understanding, goodness, justice beauty, order, symmetry

Esteem needs
competence, approval, recognition

Belongingness and love needs
affiliation, acceptance, affection

Safety needs
security, physiological safety

Physiological needs
food, drink

KNOW YOUR MASLOW'S HIERARCHY OF NEEDS

Maslow's Hierarchy of Needs is a well-known theory in psychology originated by Abraham Maslow in 1943 and was used to study motivation. Human needs are often depicted in a pyramid. He created the tiered system and initially asserted that the needs listed lower in the hierarchy must be satisfied internally before one can meet higher up needs. Basic needs were thought of as basic survival needs, whereas the highest level relates to self-actualization and living to your fullest potential.

As you can imagine, what motivates us or what makes us feel good has changed in some ways since the 1940s. Maslow and others later agreed that this is not a system where one is dependent on another. I encourage my patients to interpret these needs as they relate to current understandings. For example, when Maslow deemed food and drink as a foundation, it's unlikely he considered all the over-processed and chemically addictive foods we have today. He also did not think that skincare or aesthetics contributed to living our best lives. Since its original description, the diagram and associated ideas have evolved and been reinterpreted variously. Today, I argue that we should consider aesthetics and beauty to be in the hierarchy. The key is to know your own hierarchy and determine what works for you. Remember, the process of meeting these tiered needs can be fluid as opposed to meeting one before the next. Additionally, you can meet multiple needs at the same time. As the title of this chapter suggests: know your Maslow's and don't be afraid to incorporate beauty into your life.

While making rounds at the nursing home and hospital, when I used to encounter debilitated, sick, elderly patients, I sometimes felt strangely relieved to learn that some had dementia. Dementia had become their blessing. Their brain had gone blank so they could be shielded from the misery of chronic and painful illnesses. I wondered why an entire population aged so poorly. *How can it not be an urgent public health problem when a large number of people age badly and become unproductive and unwell for a substantial portion of their lives?* Shouldn't that be considered a public health problem?[3] I arrived at this point and, in fact, drafted this work before encountering Louise Aronson's *Elderhood: Redefining Aging, Transforming Medicine, Reimagining Life* (New York: Bloomsbury, 2019). As should be apparent, I am in complete agreement with Dr. Aronson's argument in her important work. Science and medicine are not doing their jobs when they merely make people live longer lives but fail also to secure good health, well-being, productivity, beauty, and vitality. The concept of "health" has to change. It can no longer mean just the absence of disease. I routinely advise my clients that if a doctor spends 15 minutes every year on a physical exam, only to ensure you haven't developed any diseases, and then gives you a green light to keep doing what you are doing, you might need to reconsider your treatment with that doctor.

---

[3] I arrived at this point and, in fact, drafted this work before encountering Louise Aronson's *Elderhood: Redefining Aging, Transforming Medicine, Reimagining Life* (New York: Bloomsbury, 2019). As should be apparent, I am in complete agreement with Dr. Aronson's argument in her important work.

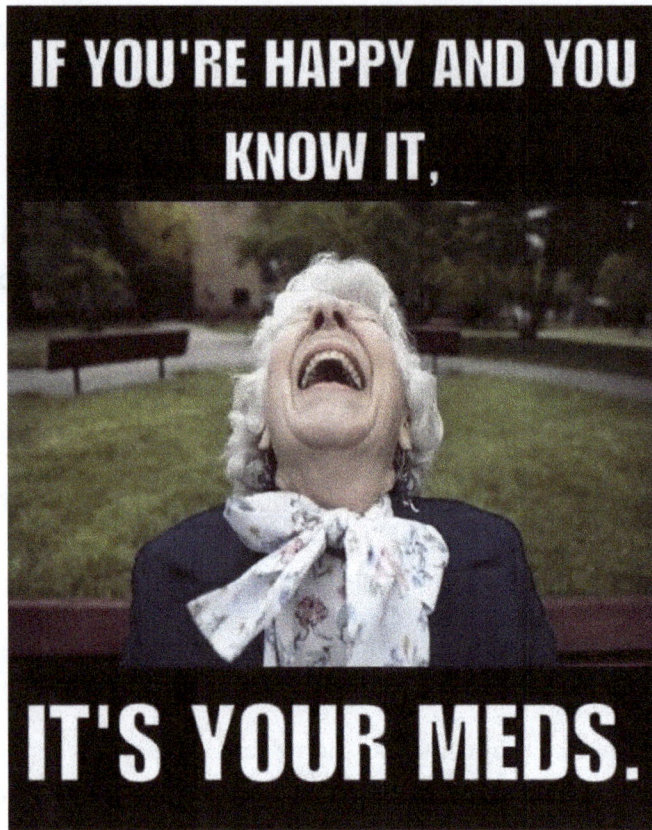

IF YOU'RE HAPPY AND YOU KNOW IT,

IT'S YOUR MEDS.

With most doctors, wellness is seen as your own responsibility. Educating yourself about healthy aging is also your own responsibility. When doctors train, there is a lack of emphasis on disease prevention, let alone on how to identify habits, strategies, and lifestyles that contribute to long-term well-being and mental and physical flourishing, which are the focuses of my anti-aging practice and this book. In fact, some doctors in the United States get paid more when patients have chronic issues with multiple diseases and are on several medications. This needs to change. I certainly don't have all the answers on how to reorient the healthcare system to prioritize lifelong well-being. I don't have all the knowledge, skills, and means to offer every service myself; however, I do have some important insights to share, rooted in my own practices and life experiences.

Initially, I experimented with anti-aging and aesthetics simply to help myself. I didn't have extra money to spend in a plastic surgeon's office to prevent my own wrinkles. Still, I believed wrinkles would totally destroy my fragile self-esteem, so I fought back. I felt so wonderful when I first got my Botox treatment and my wrinkles smoothed out. Thank you, Lord—at least my face looked cute! And that's when I began to discover that, if I could feel so much better after anti-aging treatments, other people could feel this benefit, too. In 2012, after acquiring my new skills, I opened my wellness center and started to offer patients procedures.

> "LET'S DO WHAT WE LOVE
> AND DO A LOT OF IT."
>
> MARC JACOBS

My practice became more successful as I became better at offering these services. I am basically a workaholic, a trait I inherited from my father, and working to improve my skills gave me the opportunity to escape the confines of an unhappy marriage. I also do my best to study several fields at once so I can integrate insights from nutrition, aesthetics, and conventional medicine. It helps that, as my anti-aging practice has grown, I have still maintained my family medicine practice as well, so that I always have one foot in the pond of traditional medicine and disease treatment.

Before filler

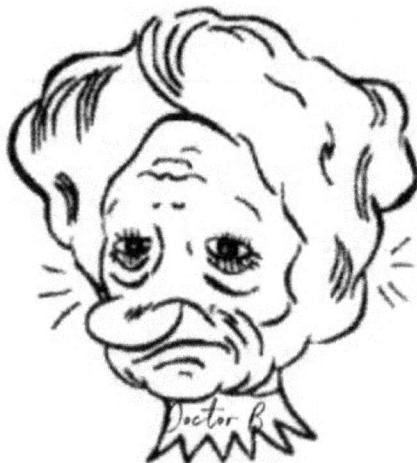

After filler

In the chapters that follow, I introduce how to take best advantage of the many techniques that form the core of my well-being practice at Juvanni Medical and Anti-Aging Center. I want to mention at the outset the core philosophy that unites these treatments. I have made it my mission to educate people about the benefits of aging better. In developed countries, modern science is making humans live longer, often by 25 or 30 years. Although we will live longer, most of us will lose energy, suffer from disease, and see our memory and mental functioning decline long before we die, likely by our late 70s and 80s. It's time to shift the paradigm and help people not just live longer but also flourish. Let's help people be more proactive so they can better prepare for a long life filled with energy, productivity, growth, satisfaction, and attractiveness. It's never too late, but it's also never too early, to start thinking about long-term well-being and anti-aging. In fact, the two go hand in hand.

THE ARC OF MENTAL AWARENESS:
FROM KARDASHIANS TO YUVAL HARARI TO JEFFREE STAR

An enormous amount of information floods the beauty industry, but not much of it clearly outlines the long-term benefits of services and products. Most of the noise is about what's currently popular, but there needs to be a better-informed conversation about what is beautiful, what is healthy, and the costs, benefits, and long-term effects of different procedures and techniques. Consider this: Yuval Harari—an educator and probably one of the brightest people of our time—has less than 5,000 likes on Instagram, even though he talks about relatable and important topics like love. On the flip side, a picture of Kylie Kardashian atop puffy lips has garnered over a million likes. Even though that doesn't make Harari any less important, the impact of his work is likely not as far-reaching (especially among youth who don't read books anymore) as it could be with a greater online presence. How can wisdom and intellect go viral? Should they not?

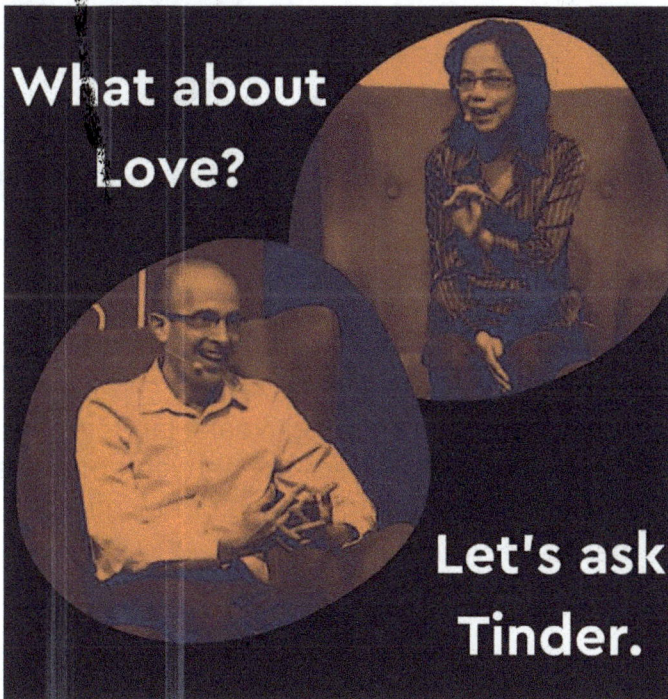

Anti-aging discourse can't be led by celebrities and housewives alone; such "thought leaders" would be rejected in any other field with implications to public health and personal well-being. We need philosophers, educators, doctors, and thinkers to enter the beauty debate so sexy, bald heroes like Dr. Harari can raise our awareness beyond the spectacle of Kardashian-gazing.

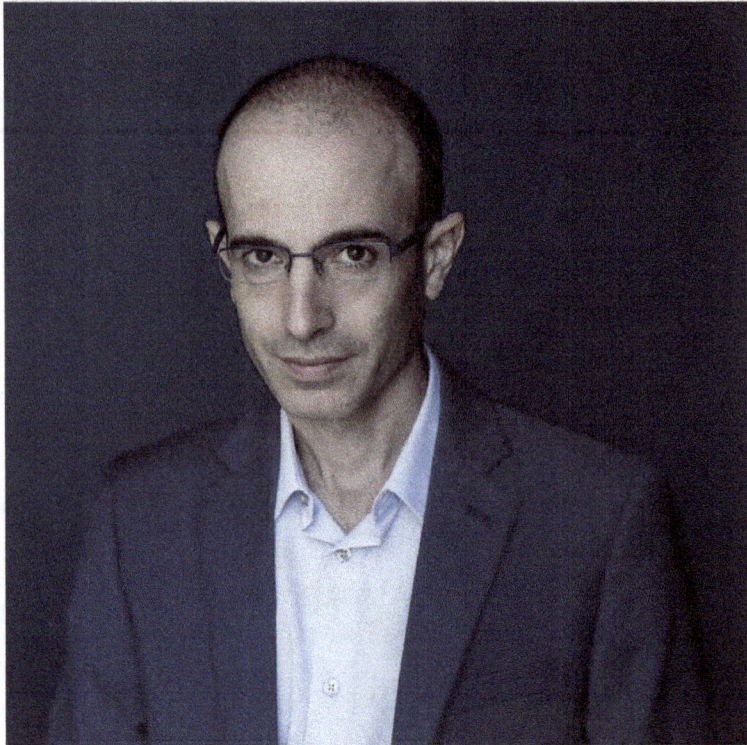

♡ ◯ ◁   ⊓

👤 Liked by **jimkwik** and **5,443 others**

yuval_noah_harari Yuval Noah Harari recently spoke about the difference between power and wisdom, and the importance of having both in the 21st century.

I see nothing wrong with how Kylie chooses to lead her life, but when a teenager is misled by what she advertises and becomes dismayed at the depressingly poor outcomes of a lip gloss or an over-the-counter acne medication, I get annoyed. I stopped watching TV a few years ago, in part to cut down on the influence media has in my life. (I also found I had better, more productive things to do with my time.) I stopped following the housewives and celebs for the same reason. When girls and women come to me wanting to look like a celebrity, I always warn them that they may ruin their facial features in their blind desire to look like the celebrity they idolize.

kimkardashian

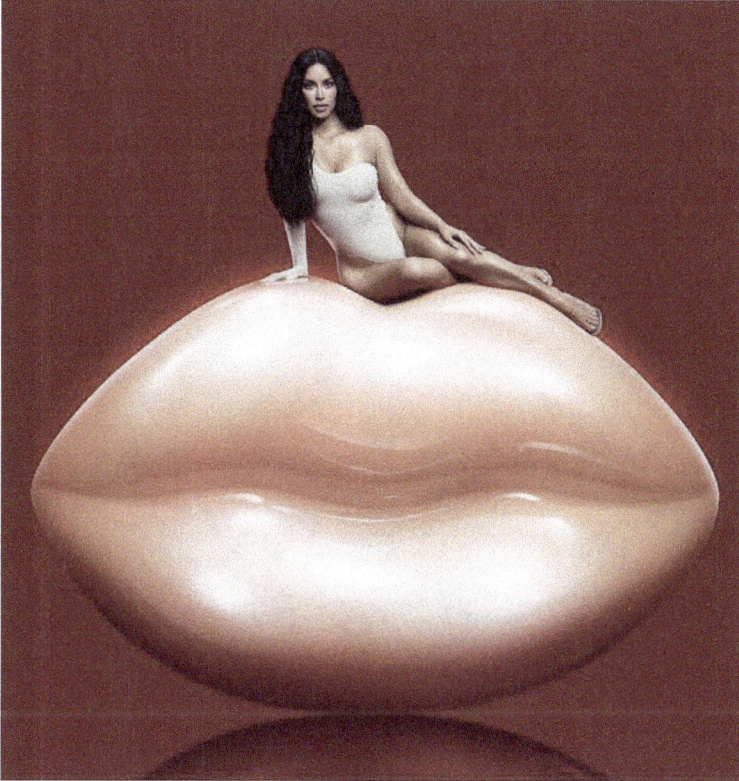

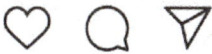 Liked by **amna_709** and **1,145,797** others

"Beauty is in the eyes of the beholder" is an old saying, and we must be our own best beholders. But simply accepting aging without seriously attempting to live with health and wellness by utilizing currently available scientifically proven methods and technologies is not my idea of aging with grace. Sometimes I blame celebrities for being inauthentic and promoting creams and potions as their sole beauty secrets, even though there are obvious signs of cosmetic treatments. It is indeed possible for almost everyone to look attractive and feel healthy. But there is no magic tonic here; depending on the approach you take, there will be several procedures or rigorous self-care required, along with a very real price tag. Either way, there's work, not magic. So can we please stop misguiding kids? And to you celebs out there, how about some authenticity about all of this for a change?

This is the reason I prefer Jeffree Star, an internet and YouTube bigwig, to any of the celebrities on TV. His authenticity and deep knowledge of products and entrepreneurship are impressive.

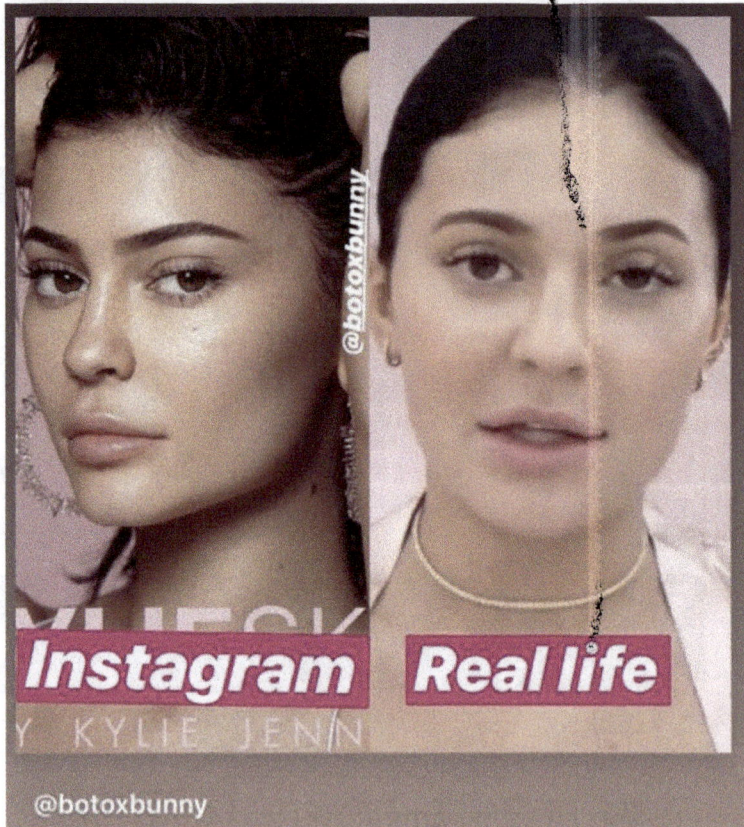

@botoxbunny

If anyone tells me I look young and beautiful, I honestly inform them about all the procedures I've had done and tell them they, too, can change how they look. This book expands on the substance of these kinds of conversations. My goal is to help you understand these procedures and their associated costs, along with potential short- and long-term benefits or side effects.

However, it's also important to explain what this book is not. While I aim to raise the current discourse on anti-aging and aesthetic medicine, this is not a technical book. *I hope that doctors who currently work in this field or are interested in exploring it will benefit from* my expertise and approach; however, my intended reader is an existing or potential consumer of these services who wants to learn and make more informed choices.

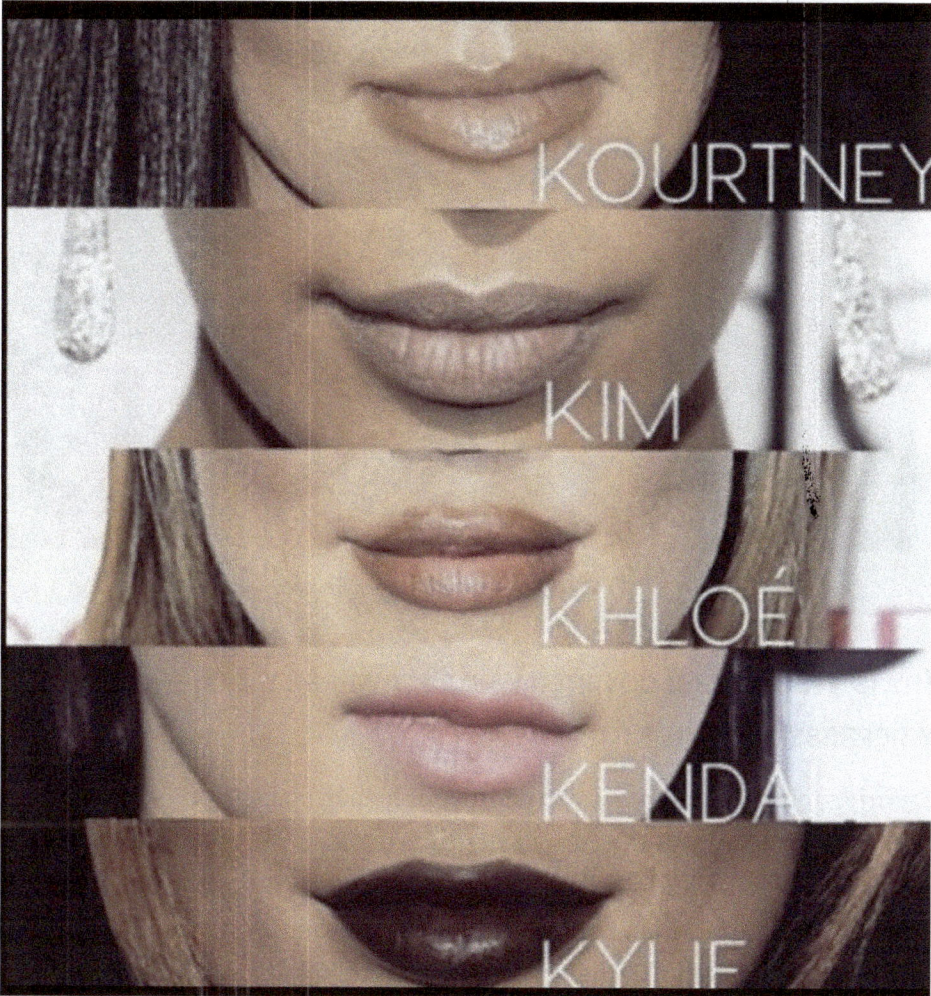

Loose Lips Float Kardashians

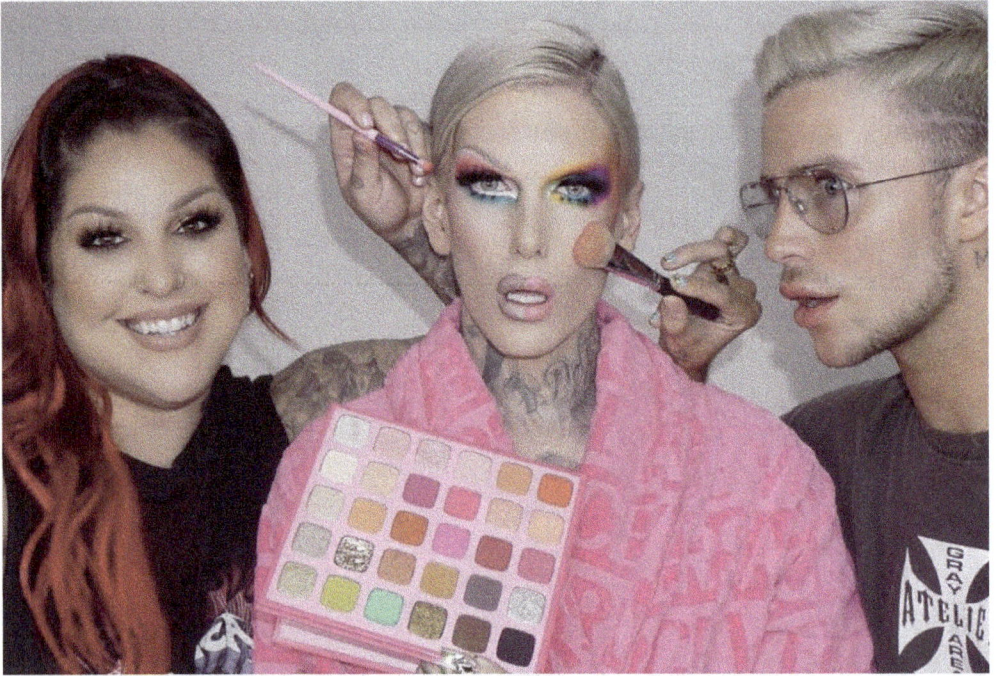

Jeffree Star—the authentic makeup star

WHY IS WELLBUTRIN COVERED WHILE MY WRINKLY SKIN—WHICH IS CAUSING MY DEPRESSION—ISN'T?

By writing this book, I also hope to enlist your help in changing the discourse about public health in order to reform the current healthcare system in America. I want to inspire you to help make total wellness and anti-aging—not just sickness remediation—major medical and public health priorities. For example, why does your insurance pay for Wellbutrin and Paxil, knowing full well that these drugs have limited ability to cure depression, but not for Botox or fillers? Why don't we study the psychological effects of treatments that alter how people look and feel about themselves? How might such treatments impact how they feel and act in the world? More people need to become aware of the potential impact of these treatments on their health and demand reform so that health insurance covers these procedures. These changes, I will argue, are important for the health of our aging populations.

Skin aging and energy decline are just as serious as knee pain, insomnia, or constipation for an aging person.

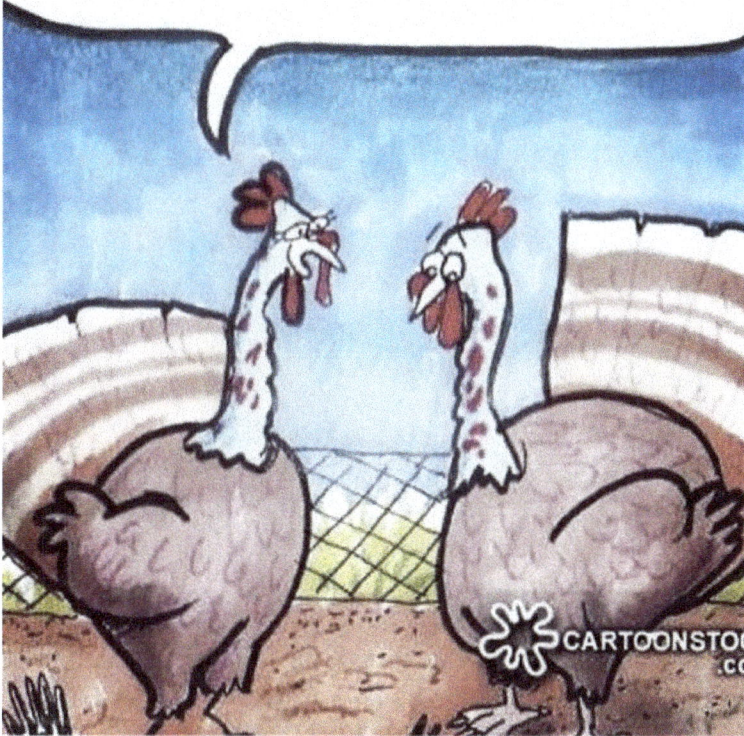

Research in neuroscience has indicated that some of the "cosmetic" effects of aging have consequences on our brain that can lead us to become unhappy, unhealthy, or both. Looking at our face as it loses its firmness can be difficult for many of us, especially women. I routinely see postmenopausal women suffering from anxiety, sleep disorders, and sexual dysfunction—and it's not merely from waning hormones, but also because their faces start reminding them of their age and their conceptions of how people are treated at that stage of life. Some can find methods to relieve their angst through work, meditation, or prayer. *Perhaps in a more enlightened period of human history we will overcome some of these associations. But for most of us, aging is painful at many levels.*

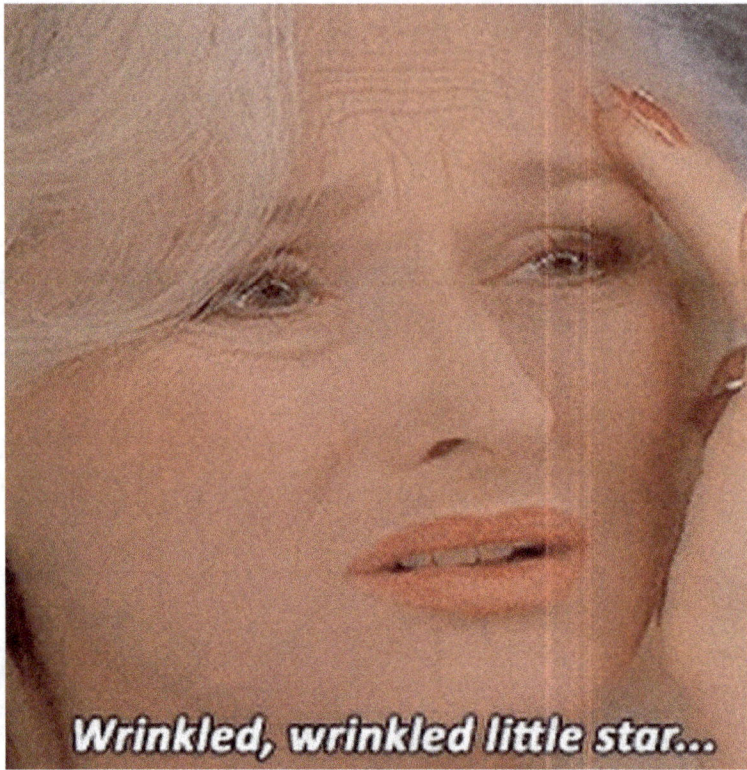

Wrinkled, wrinkled little star...

Or perhaps not. There may be biological and evolutionary roots to our subconscious associations of infirmity with an aged face. If the negative associations of aged appearances with poor health and limited social acceptance are not consciously accessible, it may be difficult to reform our cognitive processes and their effects on us. In the meantime, we don't need to wait for a major culture shift on these issues. In my practice, around 90% of clients who get anti-aging treatments or other therapies that make them look and feel younger are less likely to get depressed and start feeling more confident about themselves and their lives in general. Over the past eight years, I have seen people benefit from these treatments not just aesthetically, but also psychologically and physically. Many patients show enhanced confidence and a renewed self-conception that impact the rest of their lives. It simply isn't fair that those who can afford these "elective" treatments gain these benefits while those who lack the means to get these treatments do not.

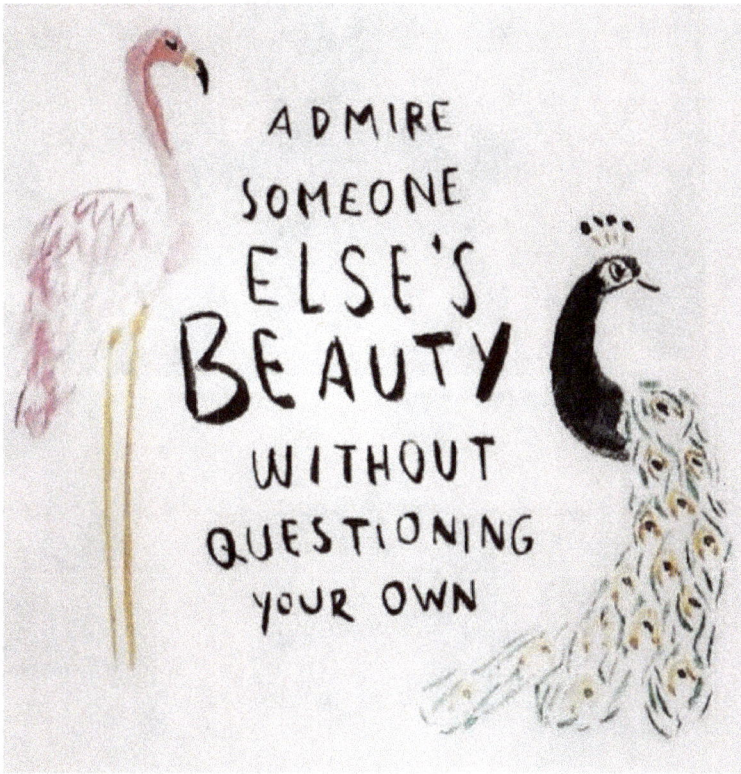

ADMIRE SOMEONE ELSE'S BEAUTY WITHOUT QUESTIONING YOUR OWN

Part of the reason I founded Hagar's Foundation for Single Mothers is to do my part to address this problem, at least for a small group of people with urgent needs who I can directly help through my practice.

In writing this book, I'm taking this fight to another arena to convince you that the services it describes are not only beneficial for cosmetic reasons but also for psychological health and overall well-being. It wasn't too long ago that birth control was also not covered by health insurance in many countries. Now we see such medications as important. I hope that someday soon we will look back at our failure to cover cosmetic services as confused and short-sighted.

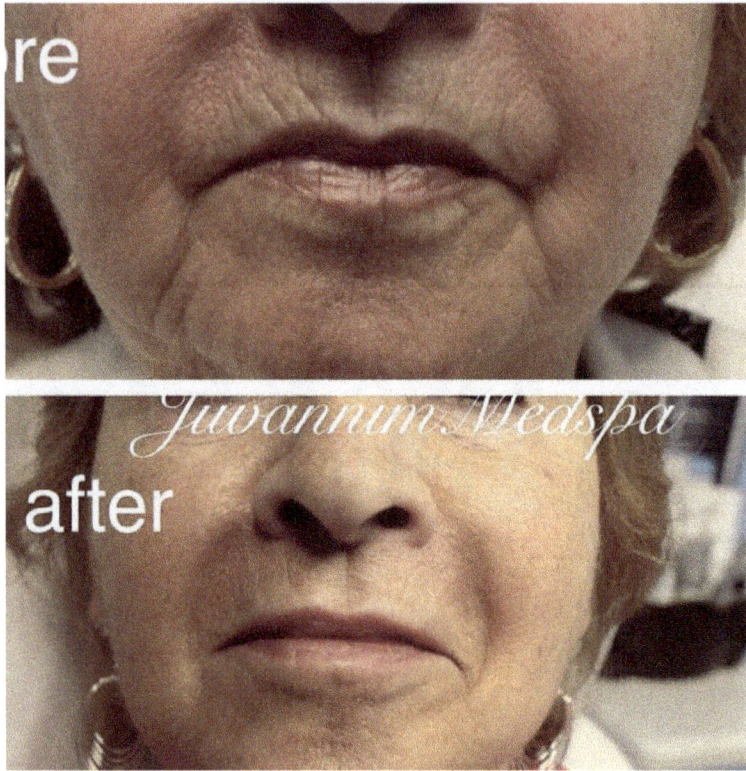

Finally, I also hope this book will be beneficial to individuals who run or own a medical spa, are thinking of opening one, or run another kind of small business in the field of aesthetics and healthcare. The discussions that follow on techniques and treatments should be beneficial to anyone working or aspiring to work in this field. Gaining the relevant expertise is necessary but not sufficient. While currently popular, it is, in fact, extraordinarily difficult to run a successful medical practice focused on wellness. It's not just that the equipment and products are prohibitively expensive or that insurance doesn't cover our services. It is also that we doctors and practitioners must become entrepreneurs, coaches, and motivators.

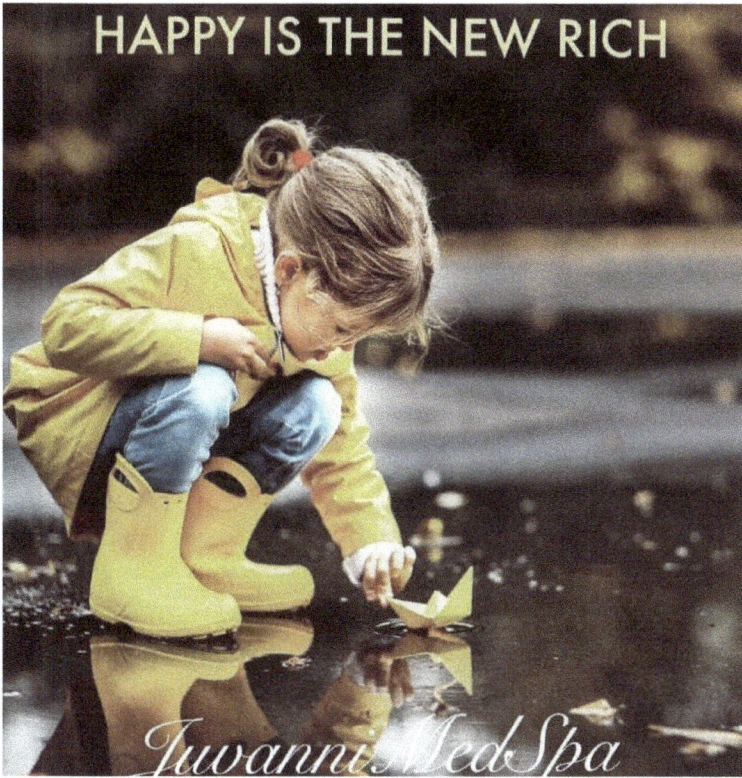

We have the special challenge of trying to help people who bring their insecurity and defensiveness (and their neuroses) into our offices daily and are then faced with difficult choices because our services are not covered by their health insurance. But you must also remember that the human rewards are also immense: you get to see lives transformed, not only from the immediate positive feedback from patients who are ecstatic about their treatment results, but also in terms of the long-term effects on patients' lives, happiness, satisfaction, and agency.

To those interested in entering this kind of work or improving their practice, please remember this work is about more than products and techniques. It's about a core belief system—a commitment to our patients' longevity, flourishing, and wellness.

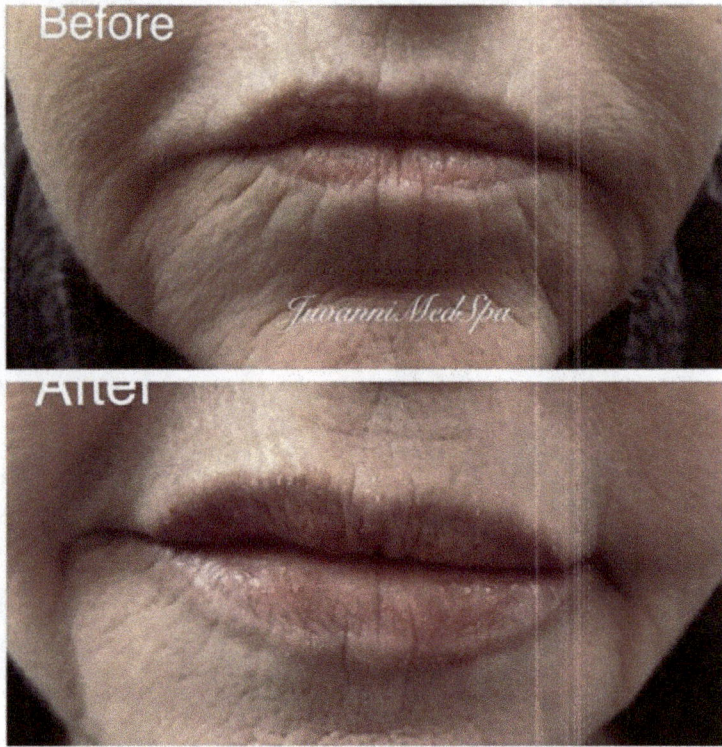

If you're interested in being an informed consumer, want to work in this field, or simply have a desire to transform medicine so these services are not just seen as elective luxuries, then this book is meant for you.

Chapter 1

Body dysmorphia—how to learn to walk with your demons

It's Not All About Botox

Before we start on this journey into the land of Botox, let's first start with body-image problems. If we don't figure out and manage our body-image demons, traveling to Botox-Land can potentially harm you.

In life, we learn to walk alongside our demons. Some of our biggest demons are our own thoughts. I always prescribe skillful thinking as a secret to living a good life.

Skillful thinking involves not just thinking carefully and critically by yourself, but also being aware of the cognitive biases that can distort accurate assessments of your own thoughts.[4] Skillful thinking also requires surrounding yourself with people who don't bullshit you and avoiding those who harm you or lead you into harmful situations.

Unfortunately, there are plenty of these people in Botox-Land, so you need to learn to recognize and avoid them, as well as to exorcise any demons that make you vulnerable to them.

One of my favorite songs both lyrically and visually in music videos is "Overgrown" by James Blake. The music video depicts Blake walking, haunted by thoughts and demons that he eventually dispels. J. K. Rowling also brilliantly personifies personal demons in her magical world in the form of dementors, magical creatures that lead your thoughts to their darkest places, paralyze you, and ultimately suck your soul right out of your body. We all walk with shadows of our negative thoughts. Ignoring negative thoughts is not enough. Negative thoughts can turn decent people into real monsters. When these thoughts are

---

[4] See Daniel Kahneman, *Thinking, Fast and Slow* (New York: Farrar, Straus and Giroux, 2013); and Michael Lewis, *The Undoing Project: A Friendship that Changed Our Minds*, (New York: W. W. Norton & Company, 2017).

directed at ourselves, they can be toxic. If you try to slay your demons with Botox alone, you are setting down a dangerously unsustainable path. Social media filters won't make it any easier. I believe the controls for fixing body dysmorphia are internally managed.

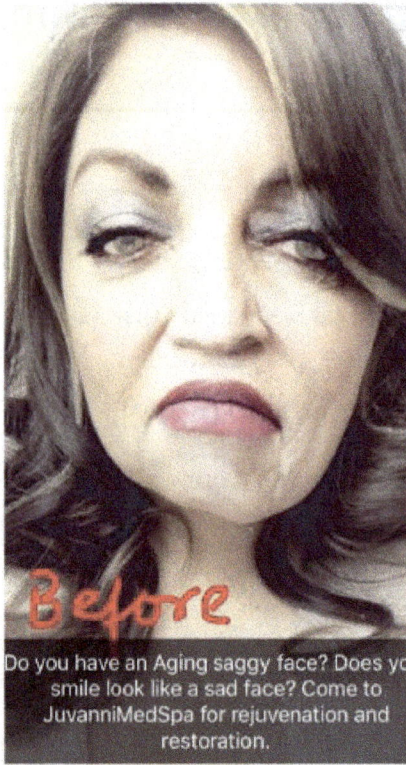

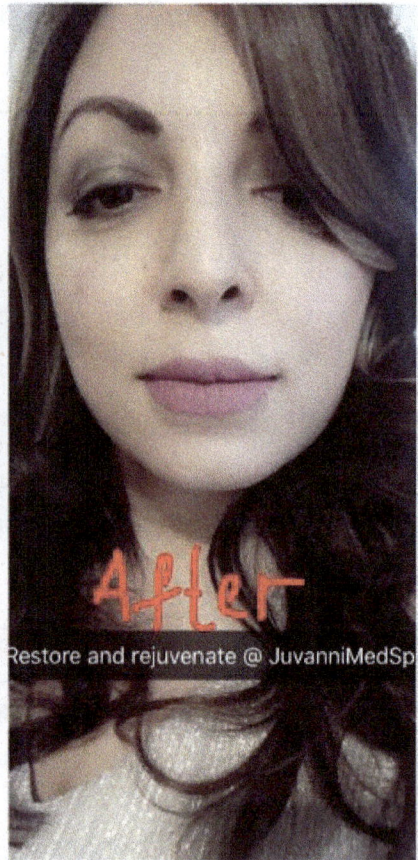

Before

Do you have an Aging saggy face? Does yo smile look like a sad face? Come to JuvanniMedSpa for rejuvenation and restoration.

After

Restore and rejuvenate @ JuvanniMedSp

MY PERSONAL HISTORY WITH BODY DYSMORPHIA

I used to ignore my own views about my skin, since they were scary. The thought of taking off my clothes in front of someone else was almost nightmarish. I had not seen *The Phantom of the Opera* back then.

It was not until I started practicing aesthetic medicine that I truly came face to face with body dysmorphia—my own and others'. I was able to recognize it in my clients as they suffered with similar issues. I had a real reason to be self-conscious about my skin, but as it often happens, I slipped into self-doubt and self-loathing. My demons were born with my psoriasis, which I suffered from the time I was in my early 20s until the birth of my daughter, nearly a decade later. For most of the formative years of my life, my skin was inflamed and turned into sore-like patches that eventually sloughed off like snakeskin. No emollient could remove my decaying skin, no medicine would take it away completely, no surgeon could remove my skin sores—in short, no doctor really knew how to treat it. Instead, they prescribed one skin cream after another, none of which worked. For years, I took methotrexate pills—on an empty stomach, roughly the equivalent of taking rat poison—to no avail.

As a result of my struggles with psoriasis, my brain etched a permanent image of an ugly "me" into itself. The fact that I was in my early 20s when it started didn't help much. I was in the prime of my life. I was starting a marriage and my career, moving to a new country, and the whole time I was nursing my ugly sores. This explains my special interest in dermatology, but also the origins of my underlying medical and life philosophy and the reason I think you need to tame your demons as you treat your skin and body. Medicine can help lay the foundations for developing a more realistic and positive self-conception, but unless you revise the way you think about yourself while receiving the various treatments I describe in this book, the benefits will be limited—not physically but mentally. Without cultivating a healthy self-image, you may be tempted to mis- or overuse these beneficial treatments.

As a doctor-in-training, I took special interest in dermatology. We had clinics filled with people suffering from all kinds of skin conditions. Pakistan is a developing country, and people are often poor and illiterate. Skin diseases were fairly common, and most people couldn't afford many treatments. As a result, medical students were exposed to patients suffering from a wide range of skin disorders.

THE PAST

WASN'T

FUN

In medical school, I examined patients with all sorts of rashes, inflammatory conditions, and infections. But nothing affected me as much as people who suffered from leprosy—a disease still present in Pakistan despite being eradicated throughout most of the world. I volunteered to go work at a leprosy center, but my parents wouldn't allow me to move to a town where people had such a horrible disease, so I agreed to simply tour the place for a weekend. I saw how people who suffered from leprosy lived. Given my psoriasis, I sympathized strongly and felt their pain very acutely. Most of the patients I met relied on their religion and faith to interpret their condition. They were resigned to their disfigurement as God's will and believed they were paying some sort of divine penance. For them, there was no way out. Among other things I noticed was that, since their bodies were irredeemably deformed, they had simply stopped looking at themselves.

At the leprosy center, I got to know several of the patients and came to understand how they felt. They revealed to me the mental and physical trauma their disfiguring disease produced. I particularly remember a woman who told me that she had removed all the mirrors from her room so that she would never see herself again. I asked her how she brushed her teeth in the morning without a mirror and she laughed. Humor can help us transcend existential pain at times.

MYTHOLOGY GAVE US LAW & ORDER

#5YearsOfSapiens

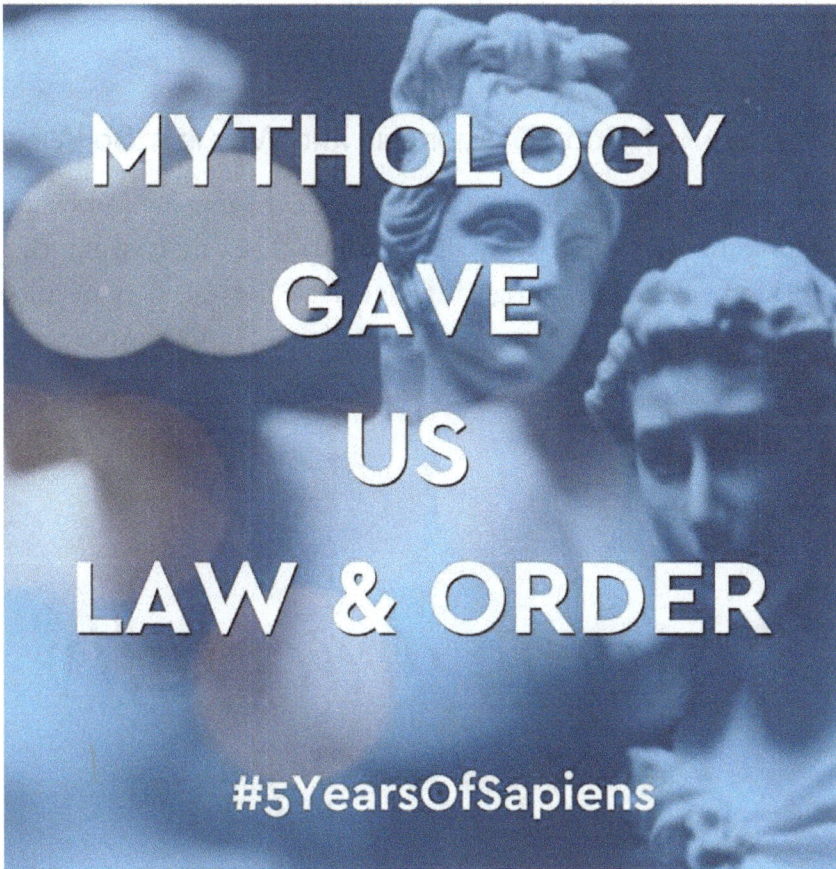

Liked by **stacyahead** and **5,425 others**

yuval_noah_harari "You could never convince a monkey to give you a banana by promising him limitless bananas after death, in monkey... more

Many of the lepers I met wondered if God hated them, or was mad at them and punishing them for some reason. I connected with these patients like I connected with my skin sores. Even though I understood their physiology, pathology, and absence of good treatment, I still just wanted to get away from them. I was grateful that my parents forbade me from volunteering there, and I gladly went back to work in the filthy and poorly managed public hospital wards in DHQ Hospital in Rawalpindi. But ultimately, I remain deeply grateful for my brief time at the leprosy center. It made me face my own fears of permanent disfigurement and seeded the approach I developed to anti-aging and have used in my own medical practice for 20 years.

WHAT IS ORDINARY BODY DYSMORPHIA AND WHY IS IT SO WIDESPREAD?

I work to overcome my negative body image daily. Even after my skin symptoms abated, it took me over 10 years to view myself differently. I tell most of my clients that body dysmorphia is rooted in body-image demons that are not real. They are just our own brain playing tricks on us. But fixing your self-perception is like fixing your reading glasses and learning to get along with the results.

Aging gracefully is for lazy people

When I refer to body dysmorphia, I am primarily referring to routine distorted self-perceptions that lead to discomfort and unhappiness, not to debilitating mental illness. More serious is body dysmorphia disorder (BDD), an anxiety disorder (the most widespread class of mental illness in the United States today) that manifests in obsessive concern with minor or imaginary physical flaws and too often leads to unnecessary cosmetic surgery.[5] BDD requires serious psychiatric or psychological care. When I encounter prospective clients who I diagnose with BDD, I advise them to get professional help of this kind. Ordinary body dysmorphia, on the other hand, stems from idealized

---

[5] For an accessible introduction, see Medicine Net, "What is Body Dysmorphia," nd, (https://www.medicinenet.com/body_dysmorphic_disorder/article.htm#body_dysmorphic_disorder_facts), site visited on August 25, 2019.

views of body and beauty that lead people to have unrealistic expectations about how they should appear, resulting in unhealthy self-consciousness and low self-esteem. In what follows, I will be referring to ordinary body dysmorphia, not BDD.

THINGS* I GET OUT OF THERAPy

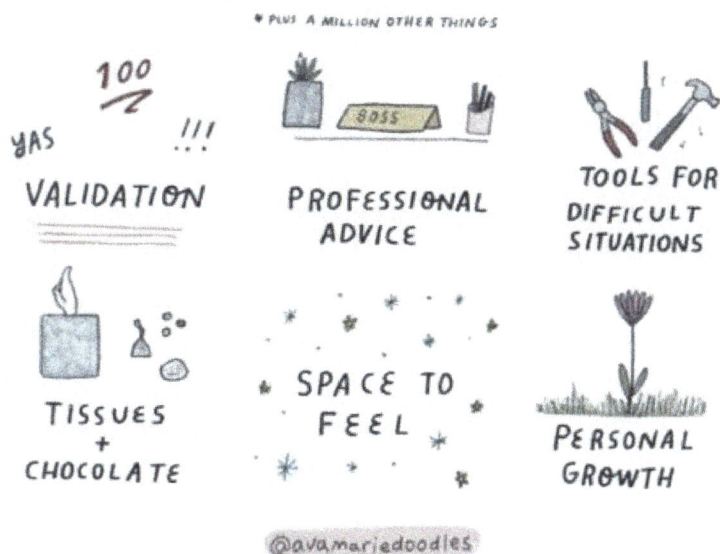

* PLUS A MILLION OTHER THINGS

VALIDATION

PROFESSIONAL ADVICE

TOOLS FOR DIFFICULT SITUATIONS

TISSUES + CHOCOLATE

SPACE TO FEEL

PERSONAL GROWTH

@avamariedoodles

The widespread use of social media filters to alter the online presentation of self via platforms like Snapchat and Instagram contributes to the increase in prevalence of ordinary body dysmorphia, especially in younger people. This is becoming an epidemic.[6] These trends predate social media and even mass media culture, but social media has made the unnaturally distorted presentation of self available not only to movie stars but to practically anyone with a mobile phone and a little bit of app savvy.

I tell my clients regularly that they don't need to look like so-and-so celebrity. Social media beauty celebrities are worse than processed foods. Too much of them can make you ruin yourself. App filters make you look like you're always wearing a perfect mask constructed by a makeup artist. No one actually looks like that, and it's obviously totally unrealistic to expect this of ourselves. Yet, we are constantly bombarded with these images and the

---

[6] See, for instance, "Are Social Media Filters Causing Body Dysmorphia," *The Doctors*, April, 2019 (https://www.thedoctorstv.com/articles/are-social-media-filters-causing-dysmorphia), site visited on August 25, 2019.

expectations they generate. Social media may never go back to filter-less selfies, but we need alternative ways of viewing ourselves, instead of seeking the momentary false relief we get from posting filtered online images. We certainly don't need medical interventions aimed at trying to bring us closer to these distorted self-images.

Beauty is in the Eye of the Beholder:
Taming the Phantoms in the Mirror Before Turning to Botox

Developing a realistic self-image and resisting unrealistic beauty and body norms is easier said than done. To be perfectly honest, it's only quite recently that I've started liking my image in the mirror long enough for me to begin my day. But most of the time I don't try to look at myself or my perceived flaws. I know that I can be overly critical of my own appearance, so I don't dwell or act on those demons, even if I can't completely expel them. That technique works reasonably well for me. I rely on the perception of some of my closest friends and colleagues to tell me I look great. I surround myself with people who love and respect me, but I also do try to pick extremely honest and straightforward people. Most of my closest friends are so uncompromisingly and brutally honest that most reasonable people would never keep them as friends. But I make them my bosom buddies. If they tell me that I need to lose weight or that my lip is looking overdone, I pay attention.

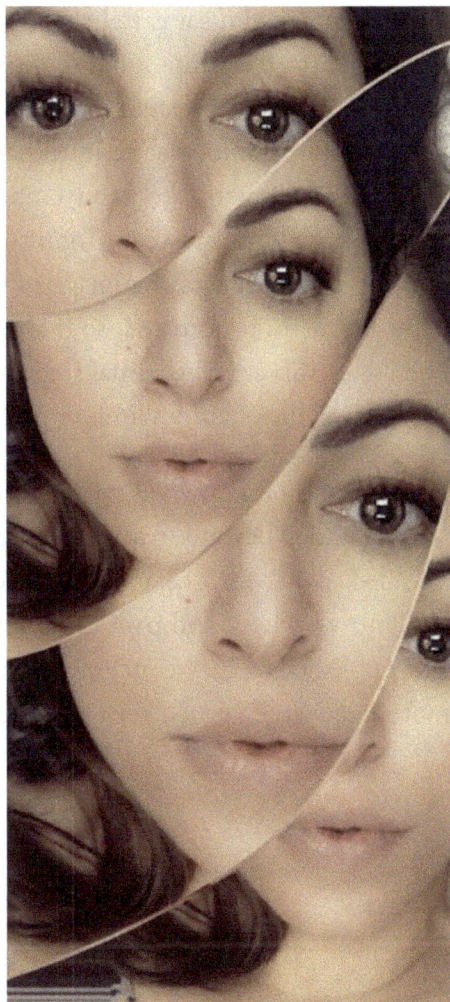

Me, unfiltered but still distorted in the mirror

In thinking about how the brain can both distort and reform the perception of the embodied self, I want to take a brief detour into the work of Dr. Subramanian Ramachandran. He is an Indian American neuroscientist and is widely known for his contributions to behavioral neurology, including the invention of the mirror box. Anyone with body dysmorphia must read his book *Phantoms in the Brain: Probing the Mysteries of the Human Mind*, which he co-authored with the *New York Times'* Sandra Blakeslee.[7] In it, they discuss neurophysiology and neuropsychology through case studies of people with neurological disorders.

---

[7] V.S. Ramachandran and Sandra Blakeslee, *Phantoms in the Brain: Probing the Mysteries of the Human Mind,* (New York: William Morrow Paperbacks, 1999).

Ramachandran's mirror box is an ingenious way to help people with phantom limb pain, a disorder where patients continue to feel sensation, especially pain, in a limb long after it has been amputated. A patient places the intact limb into one side of a mirror box and the side of the body with the amputated limb with residual pain into the other. The patient then looks at the mirror on the side with the good limb and tells their brain to make symmetrical movements using both limbs, as we do, for instance, when we clap our hands. Thanks to the mirror setup, the subject sees the image of the good hand moving on the side of the body where the amputation occurred, so it appears as if the phantom limb is also moving. Through the use of this artificial visual feedback it becomes possible for the patient to will the mind to "move" the phantom limb into a less painful position.

The wider use of mirrors in this way is known as mirror therapy or mirror visual feedback (MVF). Mirror therapy has expanded beyond treating phantom limb pain to the treatment of other kinds of one-sided pain, for instance, in stroke patients suffering from hemiparesis, or one-sided limb weakness, and pain in patients with chronic regional pain syndrome. A review article published in 2016 concluded that "mirror therapy, is a valuable method for enhancing motor recovery in post-stroke hemiparesis."[8]

[8] Arya, KN1,"Underlying neural mechanisms of mirror therapy: Implications for motor rehabilitation in stroke," *Neurol India*. 2016 Jan-Feb;64(1):38-44. doi: 10.4103/0028-3886.173622.

drnaomi1
Sydney, Australia

···

When you look at your reflection and wonder how your face mask didn't fix the past weekends 48 hours of no sleep, alcohol and toxic eating

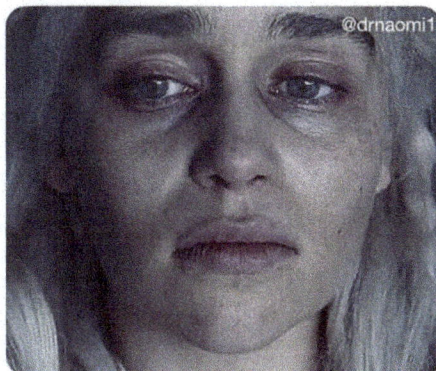

@drnaomi1

Liked by **botoxbunny** and **2,443 others**

The effectiveness of mirror therapy continues to be evaluated, and further research with better methodology is still needed. It is my still-untested hypothesis that mirror therapy and approaches inspired by it can be adapted to treat body dysmorphia when used by a psychologist who understands this condition. But for many people suffering from ordinary body dysmorphia, literal mirror therapy may not be necessary or fruitful. In my family medical office, clients with body dysmorphia are only treated with referrals to a psychologist, or a psychiatrist if the condition is so severe that they need medication. But others come to my spa and anti-aging clinic, and I meet them with the most brutally honest assessment that I can give. I become the mirror that corrects the way their brain has distorted their self-understanding. And then I do my best to help them see themselves in the mirror differently, to begin to unlearn the ways they looked at themselves before and relearn through the alternative lens of my eyes.[9]

---

[9] My thinking about how self-perception can affect your health is informed by David Eagleman's important work on the human brain. For an overview, see David Eagleman, *The Brain: The Story of You*, (New York: Vintage, Reprint edition, March 7, 2017)

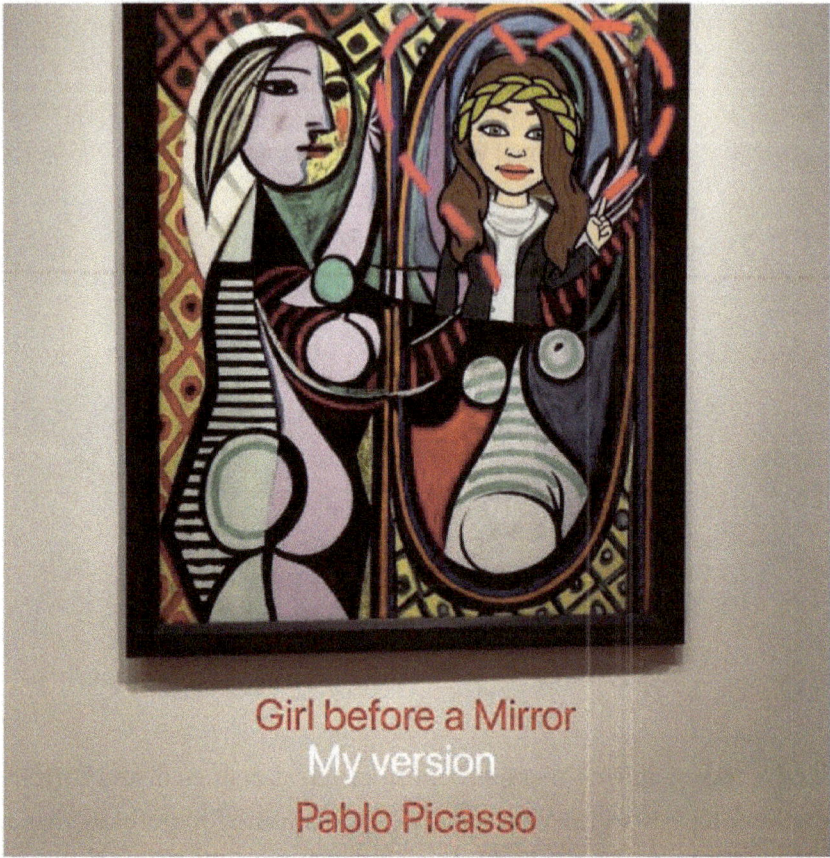

Girl before a Mirror
My version
Pablo Picasso

There's more than one True Mirror.[10]

Of course, not everyone can come to my office in New York and be treated with my verbal mirror therapy. Fortunately, there are plenty of other options. Cognitive behavioral therapy (CBT) has shown some promise in addressing BDD, so there is strong reason to believe that CBT can effectively treat more routine, less debilitating forms of body dysmorphia. Recognizing that our culture is polluted with unrealistic beauty norms and that social media and the use of filters is further distorting our perception and amplifying these pressures is a start. Thinking skillfully, slowly, carefully, and critically about what we want to accomplish through the use of Botox and other aesthetic medical procedures and whether our aims are realistic and healthy are other crucial steps. We also need to recognize that our brains may resist these efforts, since we have internalized unrealistic and unhealthy expectations long before we developed the ability to think skillfully and critically about them. We also need to surround ourselves with people who assist and

---

[10] See: **https://www.truemirror.com/**

support us in this struggle, who affirm us and encourage us to develop and maintain reasonable, healthy goals and expectations.

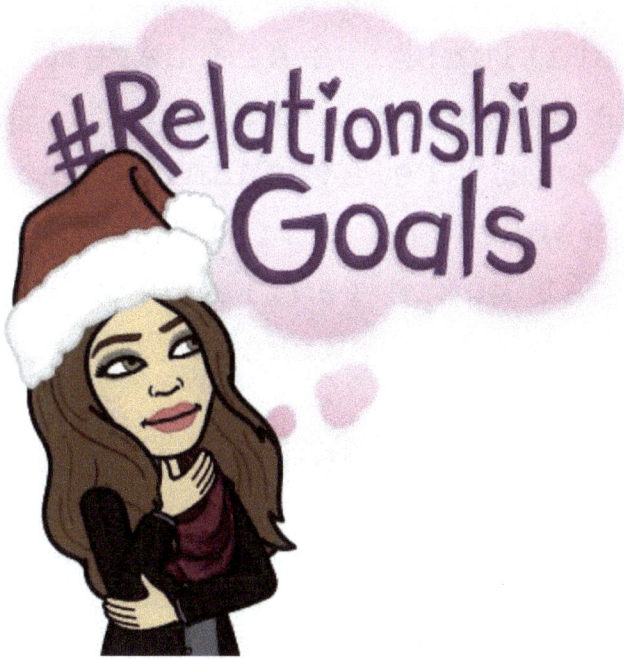

All of this should be done before you enter Botox-Land, so that if and when you choose to enter the world of aesthetic medicine, you do so for the right reasons. I am absolutely convinced that the tools available in this world can be used in ways that contribute to your well-being and vitality—if you use them in the right way. This requires, among other things, finding the right practitioner: a doctor who does not cater to or encourage unrealistic expectations or body dysmorphia, and who, instead, guides you in determining how to use aesthetic medicine responsibly. Such a doctor can be part of your team alongside friends, loved ones, and peers. Without reasonable expectations, skillful thinking, and friends and loved ones who assist you in seeing your true self, unfiltered and undistorted, no injection is going to do what you want it to.

If I accept the fact that my
relationships are here to make
me conscious, instead of happy,
then my relationships become a
wonderful self mastery tool
that keeps realigning me with
my higher purpose for living.

Eckhart Tolle

Used irresponsibly, aesthetic medicine can reinforce body dysmorphia and other aspects of self-perception and self-presentation that are unhealthy, both psychologically and physically. Used responsibly, however, aesthetic medicine can contribute to both psychological and physical health and well-being. Ultimately, as I will emphasize in the chapters to follow, responsible aesthetic medicine can lead to lifelong vitality. Botox and other forms of aesthetic medicine are important tools in the pursuit of productivity and flourishing, but they are far from sufficient. They certainly are not a substitute for maintaining health and well-being through diet, exercise, sleep, stress management, meditation, and routine medical care. These strategies, among others, will also be covered in the chapters to follow.

FROM BODY DYSMORPHIA TO BODILY HEALTH AND SELF-CARE, OR YOUR BODY IS NOT A TEMPLE—IT'S A CAR

Botox made my journey toward a better sense of self bearable, if not easy. I divorced my second husband at 40, and instead of jumping straight into another arranged marriage (much to my parents' chagrin), I took some time to get to know myself better, have some fun, build my businesses, and exorcise my demons. I made new friends, did some partying, started dating, and began to think differently about myself and my appearance. Eventually,

I also started exercising, eating better, and meditating. In retrospect, this was a holistic process in which many steps contributed to my progress. Botox was not a magic potion that transformed me overnight from a repressed housewife to a successful businesswoman. It didn't change me from being a highly self-conscious woman lacking in confidence to someone with a more realistic and positive self-understanding. But, if I'm honest with myself, I do believe that Botox was one important ingredient in my eventual transformation. It was not a substitute for hard work, self-reflection, and self-care, but it helped me to adjust my self-conception in a more realistic direction so I could detect rather than distort aspects of my inner and outer beauty.

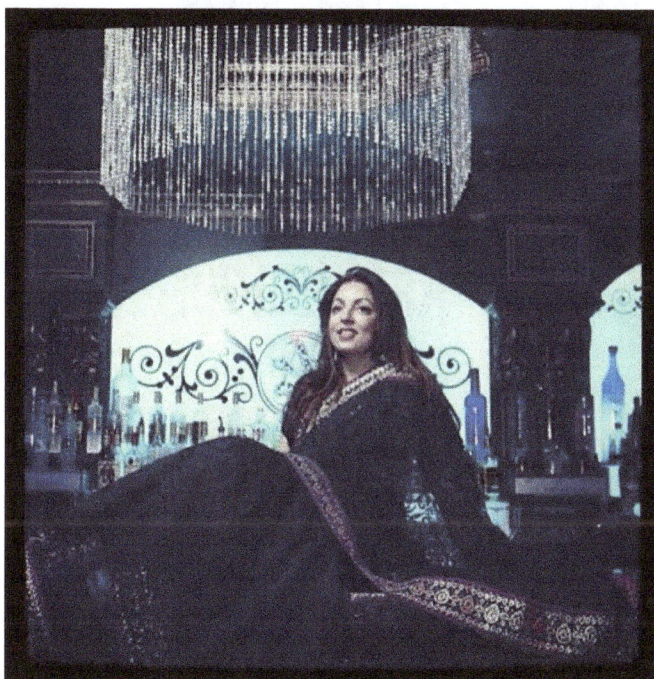

Celebrating my midlife crisis on my 40th birthday after divorcing my second husband.

By the way, though my journey took me through a period of partying, as reflected in the image above, I recently also quit all alcohol. There are obvious health benefits to this, but knowing how alcohol is metabolized in the body, I also hypothesized that it probably causes inflammation at a cellular level in my body. But deciding to cut back on alcohol didn't work because alcohol is highly addictive, and I'm prone to addiction. I had to quit drinking completely—for the sake of my health and weight and also to maintain my skin and neuromodulator-like Botox dose. I also hypothesize that our neuromodulator dose is roughly equal to our skin age (not our chronological age—more on this in the next chapter), and so I left alcohol behind. Really, it was a no-brainer. The price we pay for beauty and youth. Goodbye my favorite wines and spirits—sorry, not sorry!

IN A SOCIETY
THAT PROFITS
FROM YOUR
SELF DOUBT,
LIKING YOURSELF
IS A
REBELLIOUS
ACT

Caroline Caldwell's Viral Graffiti Art

The work I've done in transforming my own self-conception and health makes it easier to discuss beauty and anti-aging frankly with my patients. I sometimes use a car analogy. If God gave you a Honda Civic and you want to turn the body of that car into a Rolls-Royce, you may need to get realistic. Very few people have a Rolls-Royce, and the few that actually do may not even be happy or consider it a blessing. (Try Googling how much it costs to maintain a Rolls-Royce; apparently, the oil change alone costs in excess of 600 dollars! No thanks . . .) Perhaps, instead of a Rolls-Royce, you set a more realistic objective, something more like a Mercedes—still an attractive car. And, if you aspire to upgrade to a Mercedes, you will also need to upgrade the engine. A luxury car body can only take you far if you maintain the engine and other mechanical parts. Likewise, Botox on its own will only take you so far.

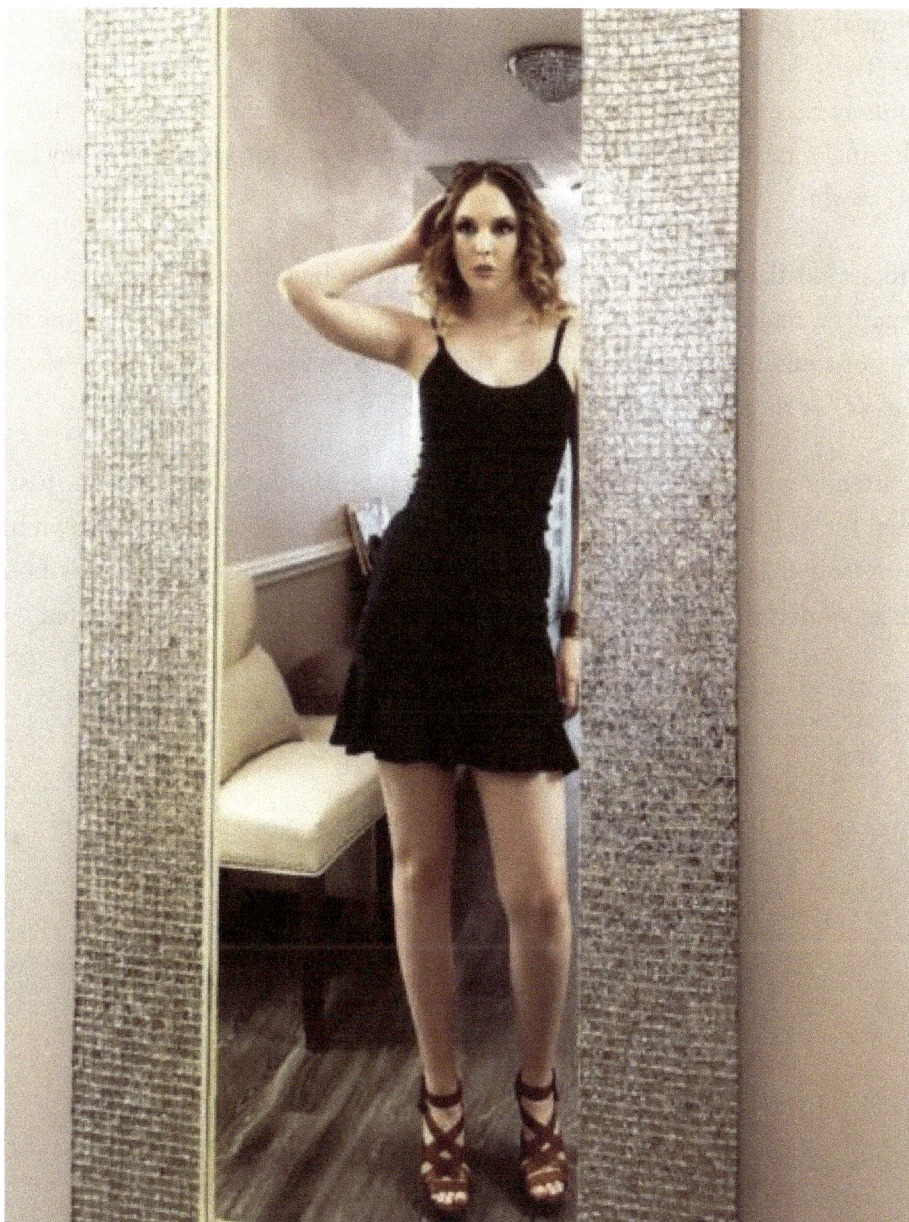

I see women who get a tremendous amount of aesthetic work done; yet, they have poor eating habits and toxic lifestyles. Despite the aesthetic work, they remain unhappy and unfulfilled. But I also see people with very healthy lifestyles who don't maintain or care about their outward appearance. Some even act as if it's taboo to keep up it.

Sticking to the car analogy, I ask clients: If God blessed you with a Lamborghini and it got bumps and scratches from routine driving, would you get it fixed? Would you put poor-quality gas in a performance automobile? Would you let it stay dirty? People don't think twice about maintaining and upgrading their cars. In fact, most will agree it's absolutely necessary. If this is so obvious, I ask my clients and patients, why then are you neglecting your own body? How is your own body less important than any Lamborghini in the world?

I understand that people can potentially object to being compared to a vehicle, but this comparison makes sense to most of my clients. After all, our bodies are the vehicles that carry our souls and represent them in the world. *Our body is like a vehicle that we can't get out of. When we get out of this vehicle, we die.*

But attending exclusively to outward appearance is simply not enough. Just as a car is known for its functionality, interior, speed, and safety, a person is also known by his or her actions and inactions in life. One central theme that runs through this book and my medical work is that lifelong well-being, health, and beauty are all interrelated.

LIFE BEGINS AT 40

So do Wrinkles, Arthritis, Hemorrhoids, Chills, Backaches, Leg Cramps and Liver Spots!

CHAPTER 2

DO WE REALLY NEED BOTOX?

FIRST, THE STORY OF BOTOX.

Let's start by talking about what Botox really is, how it works, and how many different kinds of Botox-like products are currently available on the market.

Botox is a medication, just like any other medicine you take, but the story of how Botox was first discovered never ceases to fascinate me. It's a story that reveals how humans are getting better and faster at deciphering the language of the universe and is proof of the impact of good luck.

Botulinum toxin (the active ingredient in Botox) was first discovered in 1978. It's a protein that prevents the release of a neurotransmitter and hence shuts down a muscle, causing it to atrophy. Ophthalmologists initially studied its effects on eye muscle hyperactivity and blepharospasm (twitching in the eyelids), but they didn't realize the other potential applications of botulinum toxin. Eventually, however, the ophthalmologists noticed that people's wrinkles started disappearing as they were getting treated with Botox for other ocular problems. Ten years later, Allergan acquired the rights to distribute the drug, but it was still being tested as a medication for twitching and cervical dystonia (uncontrollable contraction of the neck muscles). They eventually realized that the muscles were being deactivated, which meant the appearance of lines and wrinkles improved. As with many other drugs, the discovery of Botox's anti-aging properties was accidental. Finally, in 1992 Alastair and Jean Carruthers issued the first report suggesting that Botox could be used for cosmetic purposes.

LET'S GET MEDICAL (EVERYTHING YOU WANTED TO KNOW ABOUT BOTOX BUT WERE AFRAID TO ASK)

Now that we know how Botox entered the medical aesthetics field, let's dive deeper. Botulinum toxin is a very potent protein produced by a bacterium (*Clostridium botulinum*). The toxin prevents the release of a neurotransmitter (a kind of fuel that makes muscles contract and move) from the axon endings of nerves at neuromuscular junctions, thereby causing the muscle paralysis or reduced movement. In simpler words, Botox works by deactivating nerves that stimulate muscle contraction. Botox does its job in three to four days, and what you see over the next few months are simply the results. (The idea that the Botox molecule sits around actively blocking the acetylcholine is a misconception.)

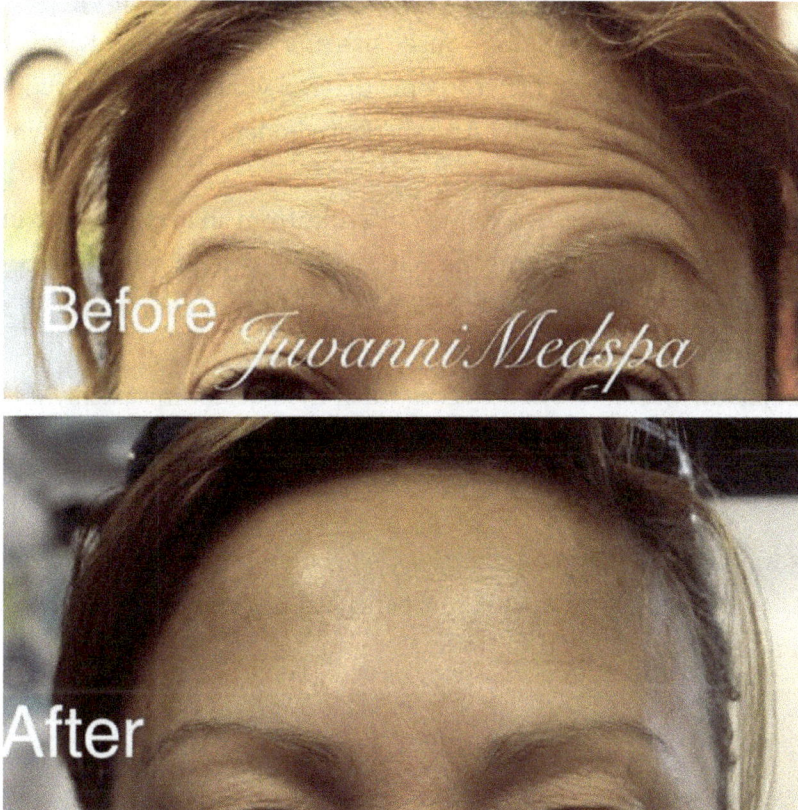

Of course, if used inappropriately, Botox can cause severe damage. Botox is still relatively new in the anti-aging world, and the doses injected are still based on trial and error. Some people need more, others need less, and only experienced doctors can best make these determinations. A scalpel in the hands of a surgeon can be life saving, but in the hands of a child, it can hurt someone badly. Similarly, a car that's being driven by a new driver can be a hazard, but an experienced driver will take you to your destination safely. Is there still a remote possibility of an accident? Of course, but that doesn't make us stop driving cars. So what are the potential side effects when using Botox for anti-aging?

Five Common Botox Complications and How to Prevent or Manage Them

1. *Pinpoint bleeding.* To be expected since the Botox is injected. Not a big deal—just apply pressure with a gauze pad as you would with any other injection.

2. *Infection of injection site.* Easily preventable if the injector cleans the skin with alcohol prior to injecting.

3. *Ecchymosis (bruising).* A very common side effect, especially in patients who are on prescribed anticoagulants. Such patients should be advised to avoid these medications, if possible, for one to two weeks before injections. Also, some patients just bruise easily. An experienced doctor will apply ice immediately after injection.

4. *Ptosis (a droopy or dropped eyelid).* Results from an inexperienced injector injecting in the wrong areas. Ptosis usually resolves itself in two to three weeks without additional interventions. A 2.5% phenylephrine solution may be administered to the inside of the upper eyelid.

5. *Diplopia (double vision).* Occurs when the injector mistakenly injects the inferior oblique muscles, something experienced doctors know to avoid. (This is not permanent, but could take two to three months to resolve.)

The best way to avoid these complications is to be an informed consumer and ask the right questions to make sure the doctor is experienced, successful, and a good match for you. More on this below.

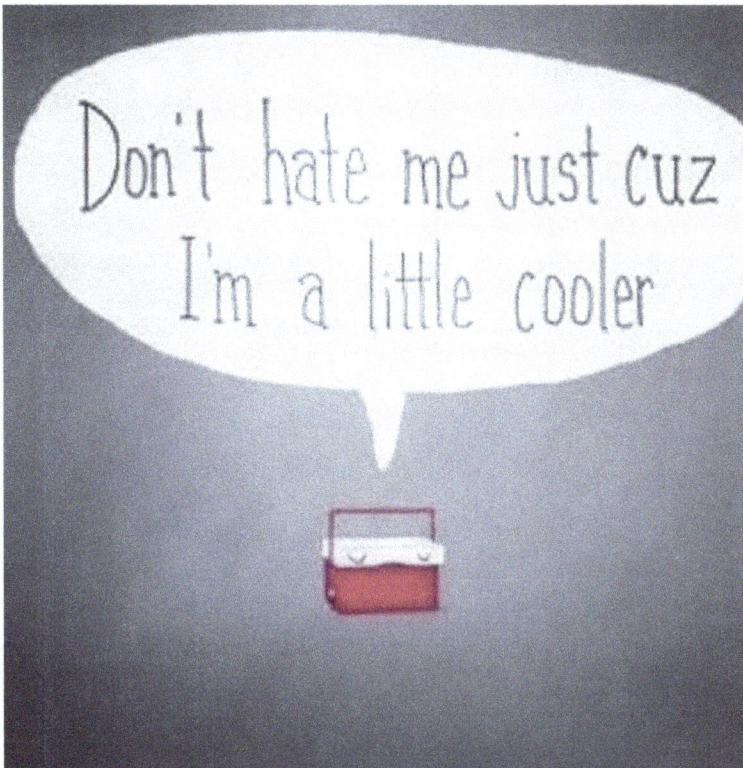

Contraindications

Please don't use Botox if you are:

- Suffering from a neuromuscular disorder.
- On antibiotics, especially an aminoglycoside, which can cause increased sensitivity to the drug.
- Pregnant.
- Actively trying to get pregnant.
- Breastfeeding.

Please note: If you have an egg allergy, there might be a slight risk of a cross-reaction, since the Botox molecule is stabilized by human albumin, a protein similar to egg albumin. However, Allergan representatives state that the chance of cross-reaction is very low.

Can a Botox dose be lethal when used cosmetically? Humans have been using Botox regularly for over 20 years, and there have been no known reports of death directly or indirectly to Botox. In the end, the risks of using Botox are generally not serious, especially compared to other everyday issues, such as poor-quality food, pollution, lack of hydration, lack of quality sleep, and (perhaps worst of all) stress.

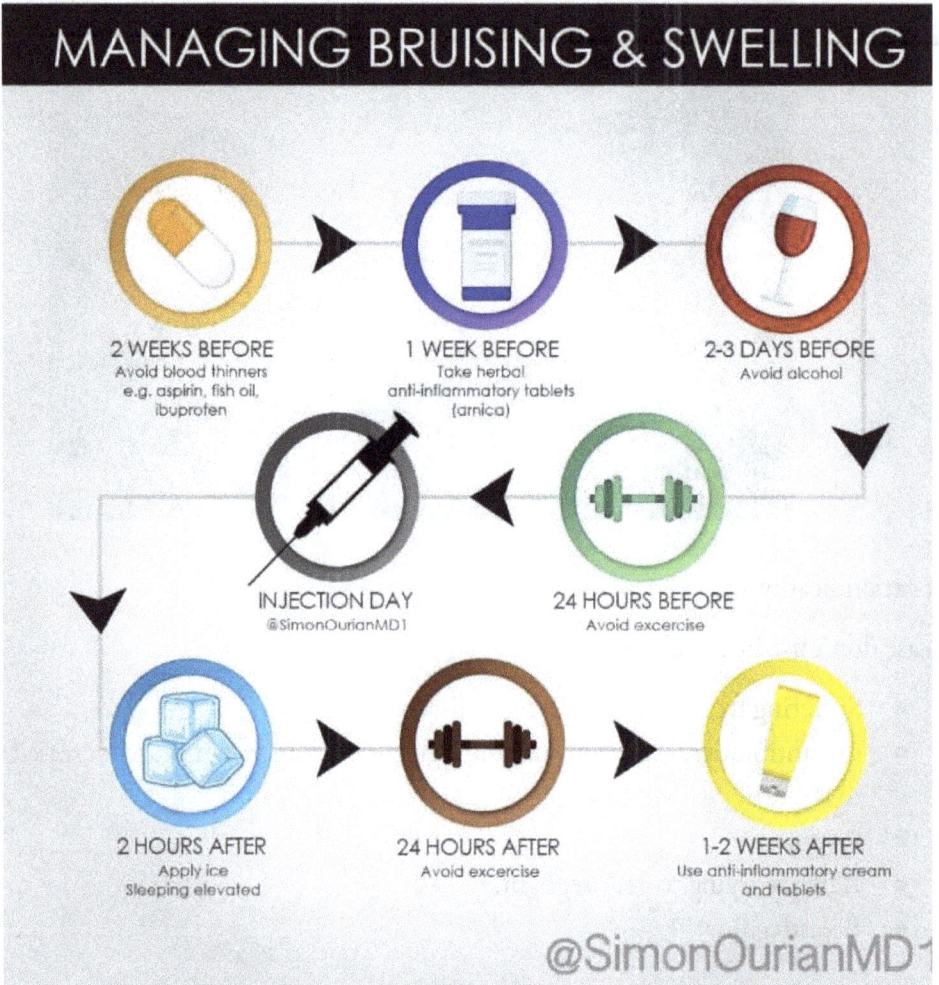

Products Like Botox

What are the other Botox-like products and how are they used? There are eight botulinum types, referred to as A to H. Types A and B are capable of causing diseases in humans if used incorrectly by either companies or individuals but are also the ones used commercially and as medication. Commercial forms are marketed under different brand names.[11] (I used to get paranoid about bioterrorism when I thought about unqualified people getting Botox from Allergan, but after learning about the safety measures that the company takes to protect this medicine, I found this anxiety was misplaced.)

- Botox (onabotulinum toxin A, owned by Allergan)
- Dysport (abobotulinum toxin A, owned by Galderma)
- Xeomin (incobotulinum toxin A, owned by Merz)
- Jeuveau (prabotulinum toxin A, owned by Evolus)

The use of Botox and Botox-like drugs is increasing. This is especially true where muscle spasticity is an issue. Both are used to treat spinal cord injury spasms, head and neck spasms, jaw spasms, lower urinary tract spasms, esophagus spasms, improper eye alignment, and even painful anal fissures (by relaxing the anal sphincter). Dysport has been approved by the Food and Drug Administration (FDA) for use in pediatric spasticity in the lower limbs of children over two years old. Botox is approved for treating excessive underarm sweating, or hyperhidrosis, which can't be treated with topical agents. Botox is also used in prophylactic management of chronic migraine headaches, and it is now even recommended for arthritic shoulder joints to reduce chronic pain and improve range of motion.

The cosmetic application of Botox is considered safe and effective for reducing the appearance of facial wrinkles, especially in the upper third of the face. It is FDA approved for the glabellar lines in the center of the forehead—the 11s, 1s, and 111s, as I lovingly call them. We also use Botox "off label" (i.e., in a way not explicitly medically approved by the FDA) for crow's feet and forehead lines. The effect starts three to seven days after the injection and lasts two to four months (and sometimes longer) depending on age, gender, and lifestyle.

BOTOX AND THE JUVANNI PHILOSOPHY OF ANTI-AGING AND LIFELONG FLOURISHING

As I noted in the introduction, I see anti-aging as far more than a cosmetic concern. I consider it a comprehensive project that contributes to the long-term well-being and

---

[11] For a more technical medical discussion of Botox and kindred drugs, see: Fagien, S. "Botulinum Toxin Type A for Facial Aesthetic Enhancement: Role in Facial Shaping." *Plast Reconstr Surg.* 2003;112 (Suppl.): 6S; Fagien, S. "Botox for the Treatment of Dynamic and Hyperkinetic Facial Lines and Furrows: Adjunctive Use in Facial Aesthetic Surgery." *Plast Reconstr Surg.* 1999;103:701; and Fagien, S. "Treatment of Hyperkinetic Facial Lines with Botulinum Toxin." In: Putterman, A, ed. *Cosmetic Oculoplastic Surgery: Eyelid, Forehead, and Facial Techniques.* 3rd ed. Philadelphia, PA: W.B. Saunders Co.; 1998:377-388.

flourishing of my patients. It is this core philosophy, I believe, that accounts for the rapid growth and success of my wellness center. I know that some of my colleagues, especially the more academic ones, begin to roll their eyes when I preach the benefits of Botox not just for making faces look younger but also for making people feel younger and healthier. So let me explain further why I maintain that Botox is not just cosmetic or aesthetic but part of a new vision for health care that is necessary as people live longer lives.

Human beings are living longer than ever, and we are just in the early stages of a lifespan revolution. Advances in medicine, nutrition, fitness, and even genetics are happening quickly and promise to radically increase longevity in the coming generations.[12] But surely the point isn't just to live longer but also to live better. For this to be the case, health care needs to contribute both to curing disease and to maintaining vitality, well-being, productivity, and the capacity to participate in the central goods of human life, such as love, sex, friendship, work, and creative endeavors across an extended lifespan.[13]

---

[12] See, for instance, Yuval Noah Harari, *Homo Deus: A Brief History of Tomorrow*, (New York: Harper Perennial, 2018); and David Sinclair, *Lifespan: Why We Age—And Why We Don't Have To* (New York: Atria Books, 2019)

[13] Here, I find myself in strong agreement with Louise Aronson's *Elderhood: Redefining Aging, Transforming Medicine, Reimagining Life*, (New York: Bloomsbury, 2019).

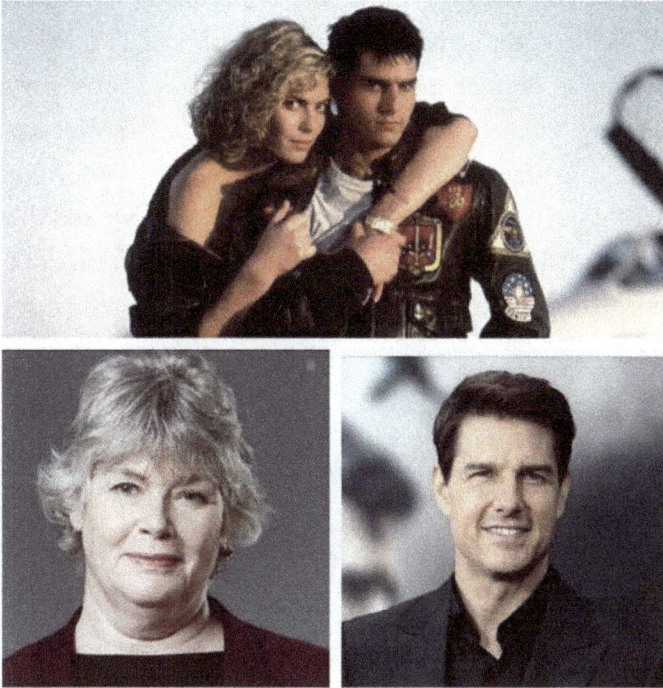

foreveryoungcosmeticsurgery

The end result of anti-aging is not just the appearance of a more youthful face but also the avoidance of diseases associated with old age. So my interest is in figuring out how many genetic or environmental diseases people who look old succumb to.

We can run into some important obstacles when medicine takes a reactive instead of a proactive approach. First, we are learning more about implicit biases and their roots in unconscious mental processes all the time. Empirical research suggests that almost all of us have implicit biases against the aged. You may have heard of a similar concept regarding implicit racial bias and unconscious stereotypes. Implicit bias against the aged is triggered by entirely superficial indications, primarily the appearance of the face and body.[14]

While we often think of age bias in terms of the young being implicitly biased against those they think of as old or aged, older individuals are also biased against older people. This means older people, who constitute an ever-larger portion of the population, may also be biased against others of their own age, even implicitly biased against themselves.

[14] See, for instance, Chopik, WJ, Giasson, HL. "Age Differences in Explicit and Implicit Age Attitudes Across the Life Span," *Gerontologist*. 2017;57(suppl_2):S169–S177. doi:10.1093/geront/gnx058

There is a related consideration stemming from theories in psychology and philosophy and the way in which these disciplines have clarified the important concepts of self-esteem, self-worth, and self-love. Let's use *self-respect* as a catch-all term for these different ways of valuing the self. Self-respect is the foundation for almost all other forms of success in life and, hence, for human flourishing. But self-respect isn't a brute psychological fact. It is, as the philosophers say, mediated by self-conceptions, or the ideas we have about ourselves which are formed and transformed based on what we think of ourselves (implicitly and explicitly) and, of course, what others think of us.[15] So if we and those in our social world are implicitly (or explicitly) biased against those whom we think of as aged or old, *we may lose self-respect and self-confidence when we and others begin to think of ourselves as old, leading us to act in ways that undermine our own health, well-being, and flourishing.*

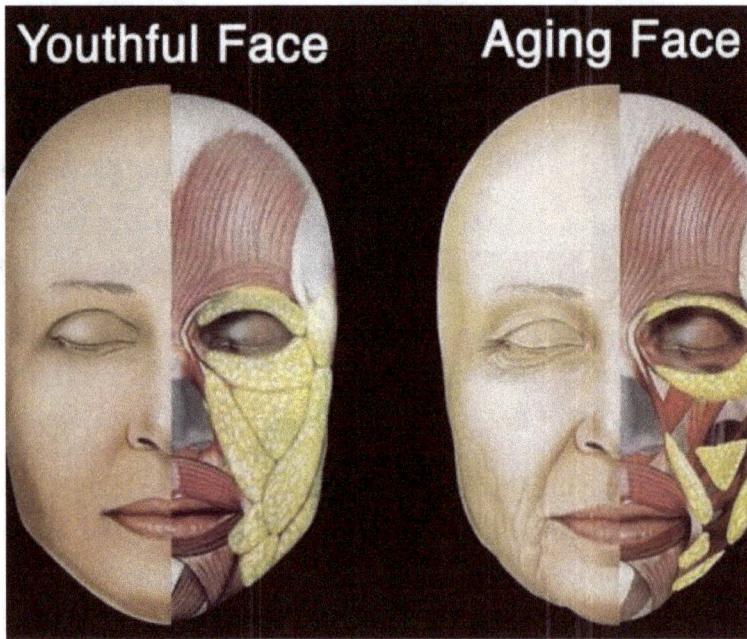

As the lifespan revolution advances and humans live longer, we need to upgrade our biological systems, which were not made for such longevity.

Certainly, no one thinks of joint replacement as a cosmetic procedure, though it wasn't necessary until humans started living long enough for overuse or autoimmune disorders to interfere with joint function. The skin is the largest organ in the body, and perhaps most relevant for our purposes, the one that is most visible. An important range of impressions

---

[15] See, for instance, Charles Taylor, *The Sources of the Self* (Harvard University Press, 1989); and Kwame Anthony Appiah, *The Ethics of Identity* (Princeton University Press, 2005).

are formed based on skin appearance, especially on the face, where we look first and most frequently.

We can bring these considerations together by noting implicit bias is unconscious and hard to counter through conscious thought. There may be some evolutionary biological basis for our implicit bias against the aged (rooted, of course, in human sexuality). Simply changing your mind or raising your consciousness may be easier said than done. So, as people live longer, it becomes important not only to *be* functional, healthy, productive, and vital longer, but also to *appear to be*—not only to others, but also to ourselves.

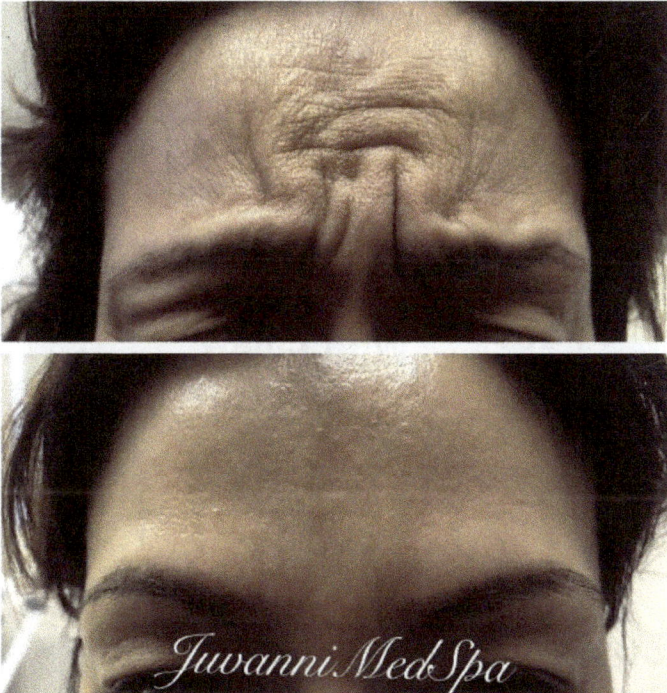

Juvanni MedSpa

Of course, Botox is just one aspect of the overall, integrated approach to lifelong wellness I have developed over the last decade at Juvanni Wellness and Anti-Aging Center. The overall approach includes additional procedures that are currently miscategorized as purely cosmetic, including collagen fillers, skin tightening, vaginal tightening, and fat reduction. Additional treatments include diet and nutritional counseling, vitamin D and antioxidant supplementation, sleep and stress management strategies, and meditation lessons. This book offers guidance on the full suite of anti-aging procedures and techniques, with Botox being front and center. All of these are aspects of an integral approach to aging that allows you to look and feel younger and healthier throughout your life—which, after all, is the most important goal.

DO WE REALLY NEED BOTOX—REGULARLY?

This is a philosophical as well as a spiritual question as far as I am concerned. One must never really "need" anything, but there is nothing wrong with desiring things that can help you live with vigor, kindness, and beauty. Consider the following Botox catechism:

- *Can Botox make you a nicer person?* No, it won't.
- *Can Botox give your life a purpose or meaning?* No, it won't.
- *Can Botox improve your IQ?* No, it won't.
- *Will Botox make you feel spiritual?* Maybe? LOL . . . I don't know.
- *Will Botox improve your emotional intelligence?* I don't know, but it improves mine, since I frown less and appear less frazzled.

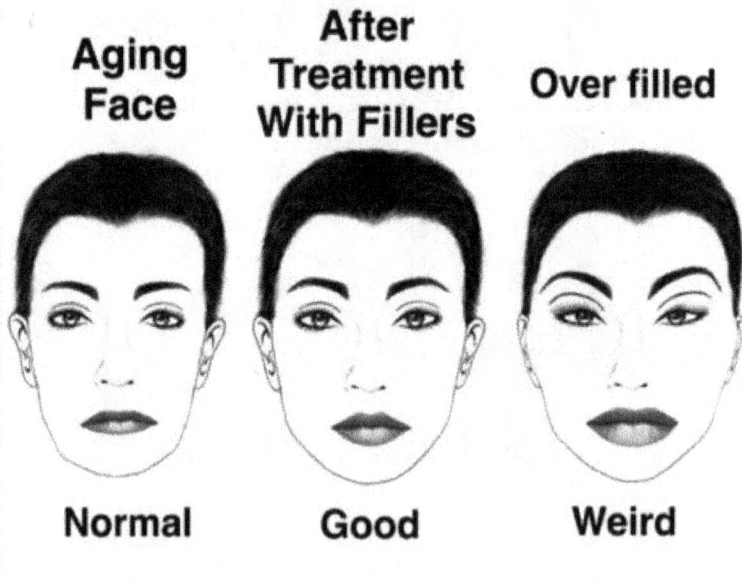

Aging Face	After Treatment With Fillers	Over filled
Normal	Good	Weird

But as you reach your 40s and 50s, your face starts losing collagen by 2–3% every year. For most people, the body stops producing new collagen around age 35. Using Botox can arrest the rapid aging of your skin in the upper parts of your face where most of your dynamic muscles are located. These are the muscles that make you frown and look shocked, or make creases around your eyes when you are smiling. I believe our early ancestors needed these muscles before language developed to convey their emotions to each other. If there was danger, people could look shocked or scared to communicate that there was a threat.

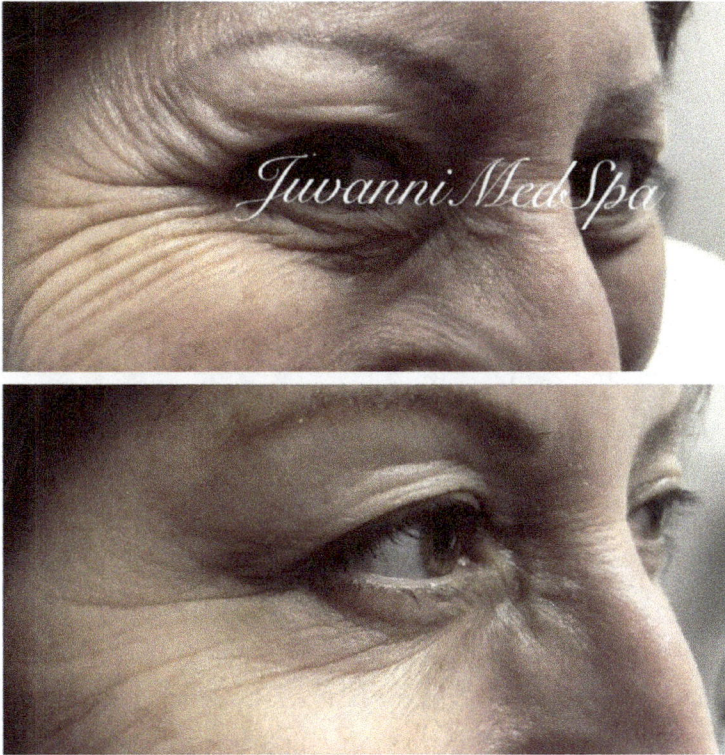

With the arrival of language and all the other modern methods of communication available to us now, it is no longer necessary to move your forehead muscles that much or to rely exclusively on facial expressions. Of course, people on average still raise their eyebrows at least 500 to 700 times each day, so even though dynamic muscles are not as necessary as they used to be, they clearly are still important. Recognizing facial expressions is still an essential part of emotional intelligence, especially when picking up on subtle cues or reading emotion from those who are not communicating it verbally. For this reason, I don't like frozen faces. A human face needs the capacity for expression and animation. A frozen face is not normal, and your brain doesn't like it either. I routinely refuse to freeze people's foreheads and suggest they seek professional help elsewhere (preferably with a psychiatrist) if this is what they want. I have fought many battles with some of my favorite clients to *not* make their faces look plastic.

HOW TO PREVENT THE FROZEN-FACED BARBIE-DOLL LOOK

One of the ways that you can prevent an overly frozen or Botoxed face is to know your dose. Our Botox dose changes as we age. How do you calculate your Botox dose?

In my years of injecting, I have realized that our Botox dose is generally roughly equal to our skin age. So, if your actual age is 40, but you were a sun worshipper, smoker, and alcohol consumer who never took care of their skin, your Botox dose might require 55 units for skin similar to that of a 55-year-old. (Note that Botox is dosed in its own unit of measurement.)

On the other hand, I am 48, but I use 35 units every four months; that is because my skin age is better than my actual age. I avoid unnecessary sun exposure, except when I am snorkeling, which is one of my favorite activities. I don't snorkel more than two or three times a year, and I use a lot of sun protection. Plus, having suffered from psoriasis, I always moisturize twice a day and drink plenty of water to avoid dry skin. Though I smoked and started drinking alcohol when I came to America at 25 years old, I thankfully was able to quit these highly addictive habits and have maintained my smoke-free and alcohol-free life for a couple of years now with great success. I am grateful for these changes, which made my skin so much nicer, and now my Botox lasts much longer. I save money by not purchasing cigs or booze, but also save by having to inject less Botox.

You should have a sense of your facial skin age and then ask for a free consultation with a Botox doctor. Ask them what dose they think you need and what result they hope to produce with that dose, working from something like the following questions:

- What do you think my facial skin age is?
- How much Botox will you use?
- Will I still be able to animate or have movement in my forehead when the procedure is complete?
- How often should I get it? What's the recommended minimum dose?
- How can I make my dose last longer?

When you have injector friends   When you don't

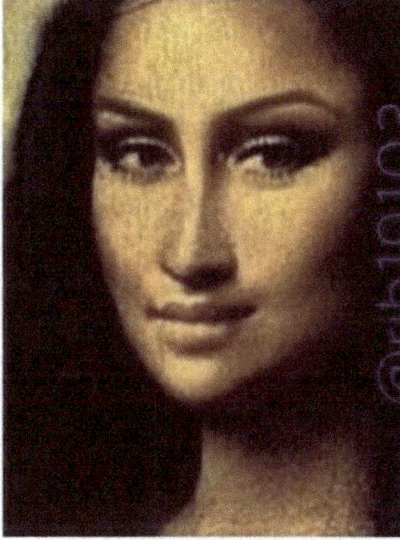

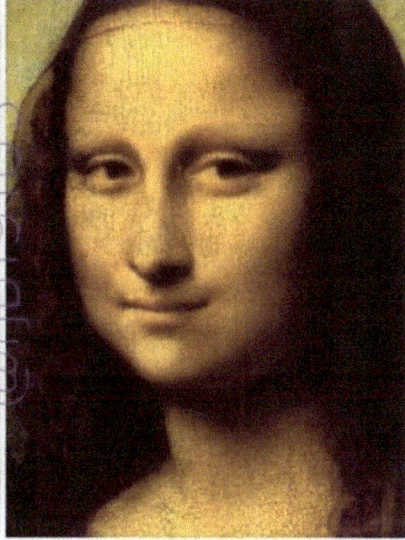

Some things are best left alone...

The right side of my face vs. the left side of my face

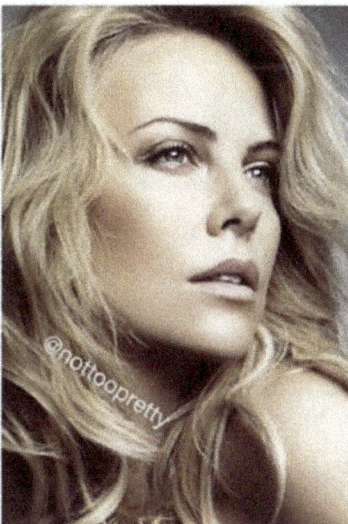

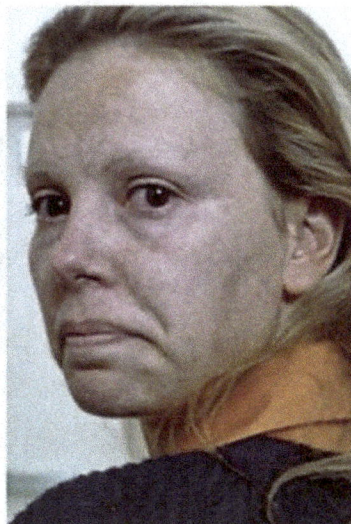

SHOULD YOU START AS SOON AS THE SIGNS OF SKIN AGING BEGIN?

Modern science is opening up new possibilities that are both enticing and scary. In the future, we may be able to use genetic engineering to design babies, and medical advances will help people live very long lives. In my opinion, the early reduction of wrinkles will lead people to feel and look youthful for at least 20 or 30 more years, which can lead to enhanced productivity, well-being, and flourishing. As future generations live longer than all prior generations, we will need to start finding methods to decrease the physical signs and symptoms of aging. Botox and similar products are great solutions that are currently available; we do not need to wait for medical advances from science fiction.

In my opinion, all doctors, nurses, and healthcare workers should be trained in anti-aging. They may decide not to offer these procedures themselves, but learning them and educating their clients and patients about them should be encouraged.

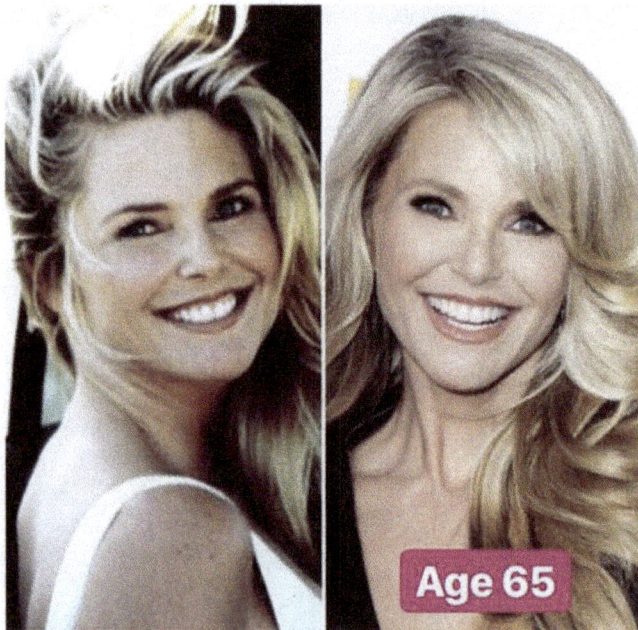

What people think aging "naturally" in Hollywood looks like vs...

Age 65

THE PERSONAL IMPACT OF BOTOX ON MYSELF AND OTHERS

When I was 38 and struggling to get out of my emotionally abusive marriage, I had filed for divorce, and the lawyers were having a field day. I was hemorrhaging money and was an emotional mess. Leaving a bad marriage is even more painful when you share a child. I remember being sad about losing 13 years of my life with someone I didn't love. "It's like a life sentence," I would say to my mom, who would just pretend she knew what I was talking about. With all the stress of an acrimonious divorce, I started noticing lines appearing between my eyes. After making my ex leave my house, life was much calmer, but my aging face was a new cause of anxiety. I also started developing acne, probably due to long hours of mental and physical work and sleep deprivation.

Botox and a little bit of filler at a local plastic surgeon's office (where I had previously worked as surgical assistant doing oculoplastic surgery procedures) was nothing less than a blessing. Suddenly I started looking seven to eight years younger. I felt as if God gave me another shot at my lost 30s. I never looked back after that. I no longer needed any more proof that these procedures worked. I knew I had to learn how to do them myself in order to help myself in a more cost-effective way.

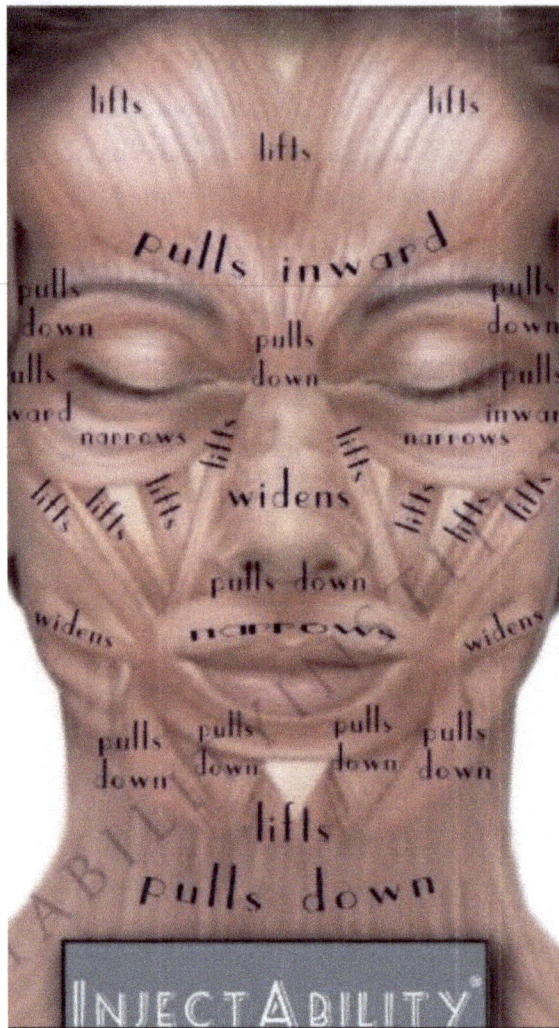

I learned all the new techniques, went to several training sessions, and brought consultants to my office to train me. In 2012, I started providing these services to my clients from my family medicine practice. I had a lifelong interest in aesthetics, starting as a schoolgirl in Pakistan when I learned the fine skills of threading eyebrows and selling DIY homemade hair and eyelash growth elixirs to earn some extra lunch money. Starting my own aesthetic business as a doctor was a far cry from what I had imagined doing in medicine. I was the medical director of a nursing home and was actively managing a large number of geriatric patients who suffered from dementia and other assorted diseases of aging, like osteoporosis, heart disease etc. Among other things I noticed that none of my aging patients liked looking at themselves. As their facial architecture got distorted by loss of collagen and skin elasticity, they got more and more depressed and resigned to feeling old. This scared the living daylights out of me and I worried about aging helplessly without any aesthetic interventions (like we did in the 18th century). Doctors usually have lackluster lives spent in dealing with death and disease. But there I was, committing myself to the continued wellness and anti-aging of my clients and patients by offering services and solutions not covered by health insurances. This is due to the fact that FDA does not cover anti-aging procedures because it doesn't think that aging is a disease in itself. An utterly flawed stance in my humble opinion. My aesthetic following got quite large and started overwhelming my insurance-dependent medical practice. As a result, I decided to build and open another office in 2017 solely for wellness-oriented clients.

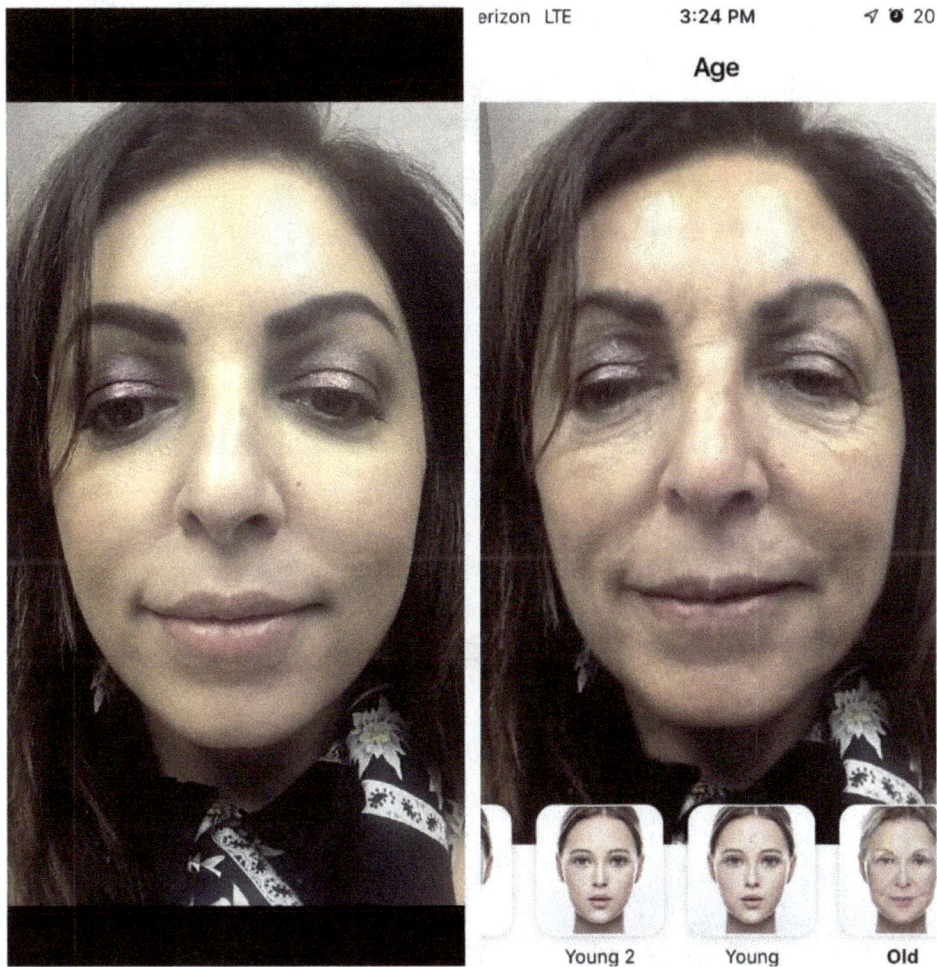

My own pic from the recent FaceApp, which I want to turn into Warhol-style wallpaper someday.

Now I have hundreds of clients who tell me how much benefit they derive from these routine services. These clients are proof that these services are beneficial if used correctly and consistently. *Anti-aging is no longer simply a shallow attempt to appease one's vanity.* It's also different from owning a luxury bag—it's not extravagant but rather serves an important purpose. Anti-aging has the potential to add several years of vitality and confidence to your life, enhance your physical appearance, and maybe even make you sound wise beyond your years (since no one can really tell your age if you anti-age). I just council people to start early like most celebrities do; however, just don't do more than what is essential for the anti-aging of your face.

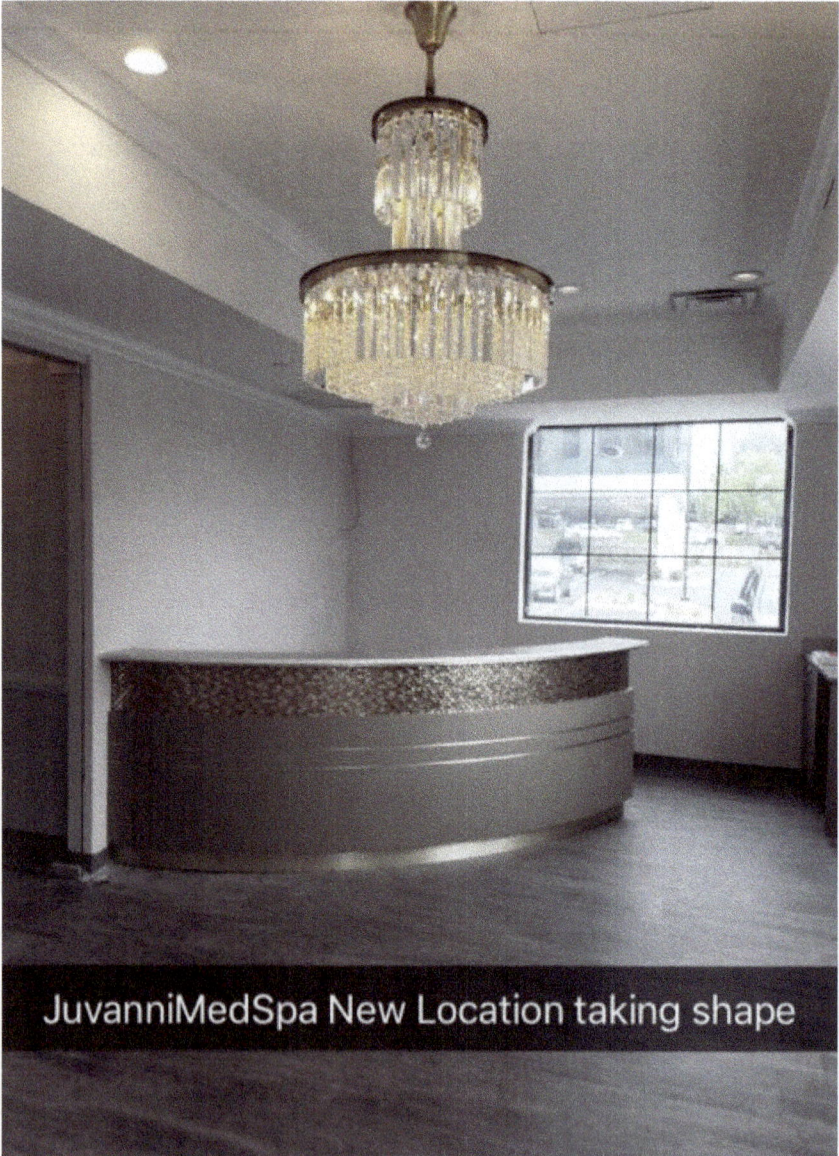

JuvanniMedSpa New Location taking shape

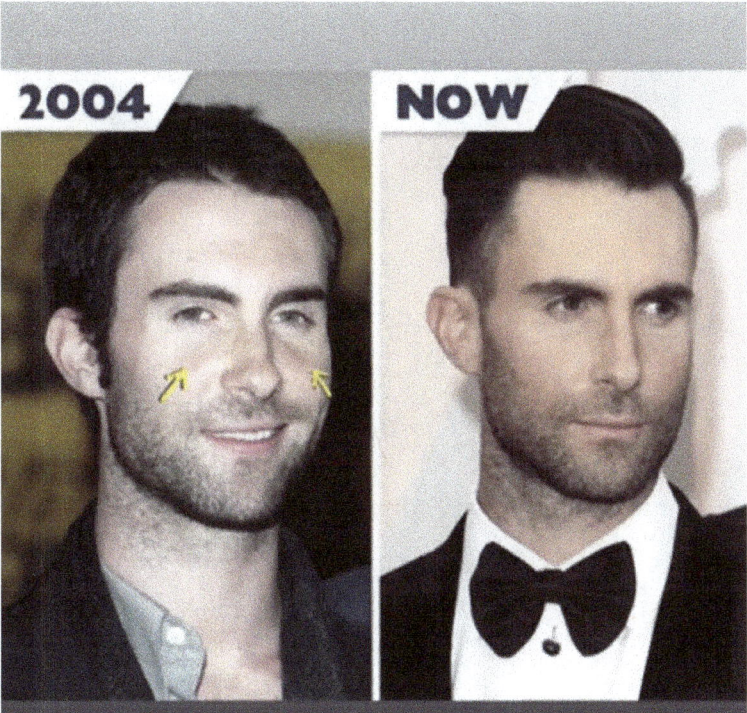

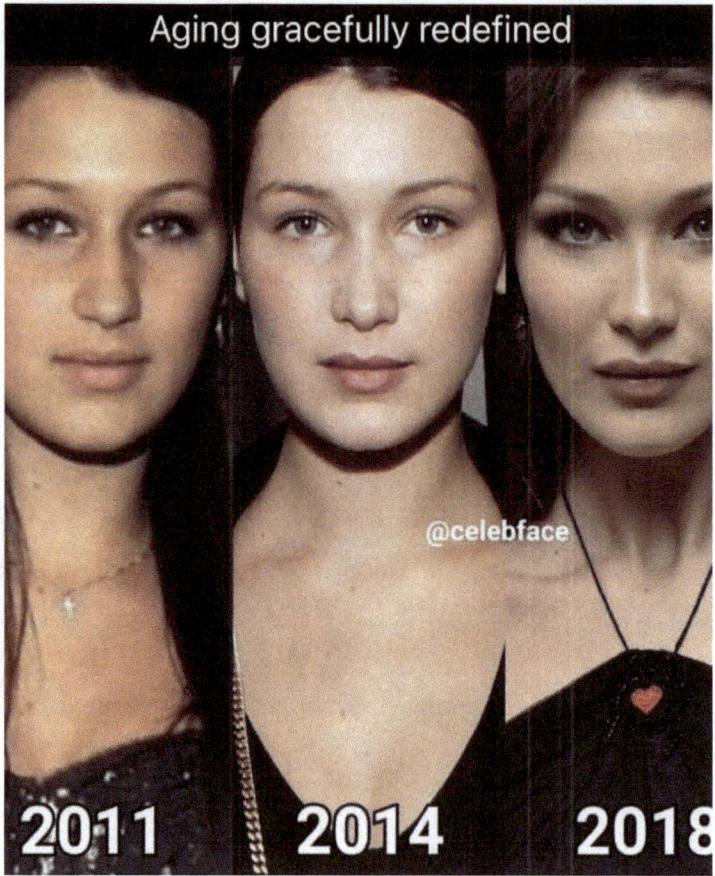

Aging gracefully redefined

@celebface

2011   2014   2018

Chapter 3

Filters, Fillers, and Facelifts. Stop Waiting for Easier Solutions.

From Filters to Fillers

The age of social media and smartphones has brought with it facial recognition tools and "improved" ways of presenting images of ourselves to others. Millions of people around the world use social media apps like Instagram and Snapchat to take advantage of their face-enhancing filters on a daily basis. With the click of a button, you can look like you have makeup on or as if you just got back from a relaxing vacation. My clients frequently ask if their skin can look like their Snapchat filter picture. I tell them that filters are like putting on a mask, portraying an idea of perfection that is unattainable, or at least unsustainable. Although filtered pictures may be fun, we must remember that they don't portray real life, even on a good day. Alas, keeping the two straight isn't always easy.

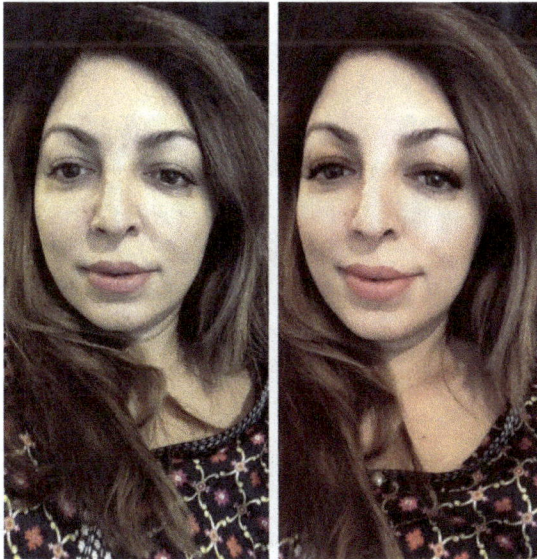

Me before and after a Snapchat total makeup filter

Botox can't be used for all your wrinkle needs. Botox, as explained in the previous chapter, is purified bacteria that relaxes or freezes your muscles to decrease the appearance of wrinkles. But dermal fillers are also a very big part of reducing face aging. Both Botox and dermal fillers are minimally invasive, which basically means that their application doesn't involve surgery. (They're given via fine injections.) Dermal fillers, also known as soft tissue fillers, are designed to be injected beneath the skin to add volume and fullness to areas that have thinned out due to aging. The thinning of the face as we age is most common in cheeks, lips, and areas around the mouth.

Substances commonly used in dermal fillers include:

- *Calcium hydroxylapatite*, a mineral-like compound found in bones.
- *Hyaluronic acid*, which is found naturally in some fluids and tissues in the body and adds plumpness to the skin.
- *Polyalkylimide*, a transparent gel compatible with the body.
- *Polylactic acid*, which stimulates the skin to make more collagen.
- *Polymethyl-methacrylate microspheres*, a semi-permanent filler.

Widely used trade names for FDA-approved hyaluronic acid and other dermal fillers are:

- Juvederm—Voluma, Vollure, Ultra, Ultra Plus, and Volbella
- Restylane—Defyne (also known as Perlane in Europe), Refyne, Silk, and Lyft
- Radiesse
- Belotero Balance
- Sculptra
- Bellafill

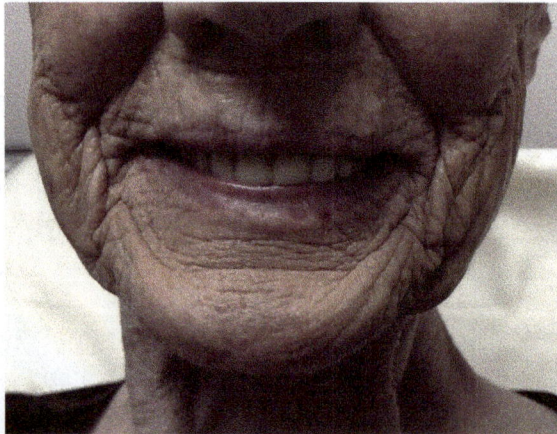

The static wrinkles around the mouth and along the cheeks usually result from the loss of collagen and elasticity in the skin. We need to move our mouth to speak and eat, so some of these muscles should never be Botoxed. Instead, the volume loss that occurs with regular aging can be reversed or corrected with dermal fillers. I prefer some fillers over others and for different parts of the face. Best practices can vary from person to person according to skin type, facial structure, and age. For this reason, it is absolutely essential that the person injecting you must be well trained and have good aesthetic sensibilities.

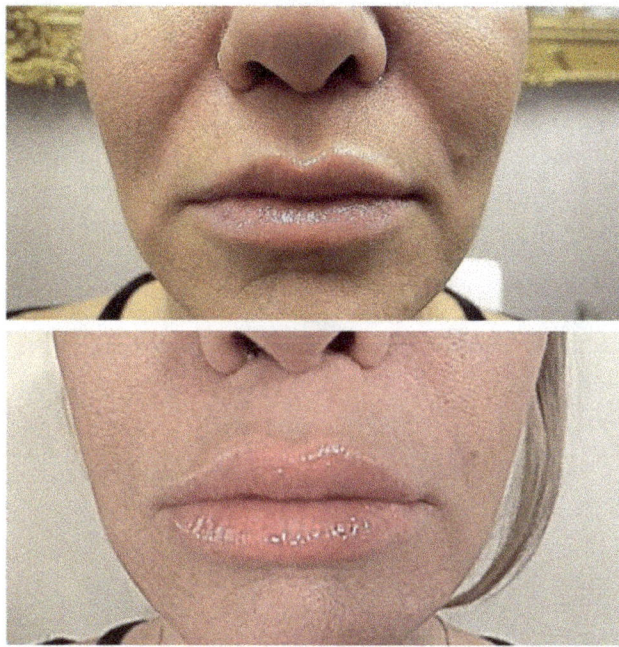

WHAT CAN DERMAL FILLERS DO FOR YOU?

Different types of dermal fillers are designed to treat varying signs of aging. They can be used to:

- Plump up thinning lips.
- Decrease under-eye shadows and to prevent under-eye skin laxity via volume restoration.
- Improve the appearance of recessed acne scars.
- Restore volume in the temples.
- Restore volume in the hollows under the cheekbone.
- Reduce static wrinkles around the lower face.

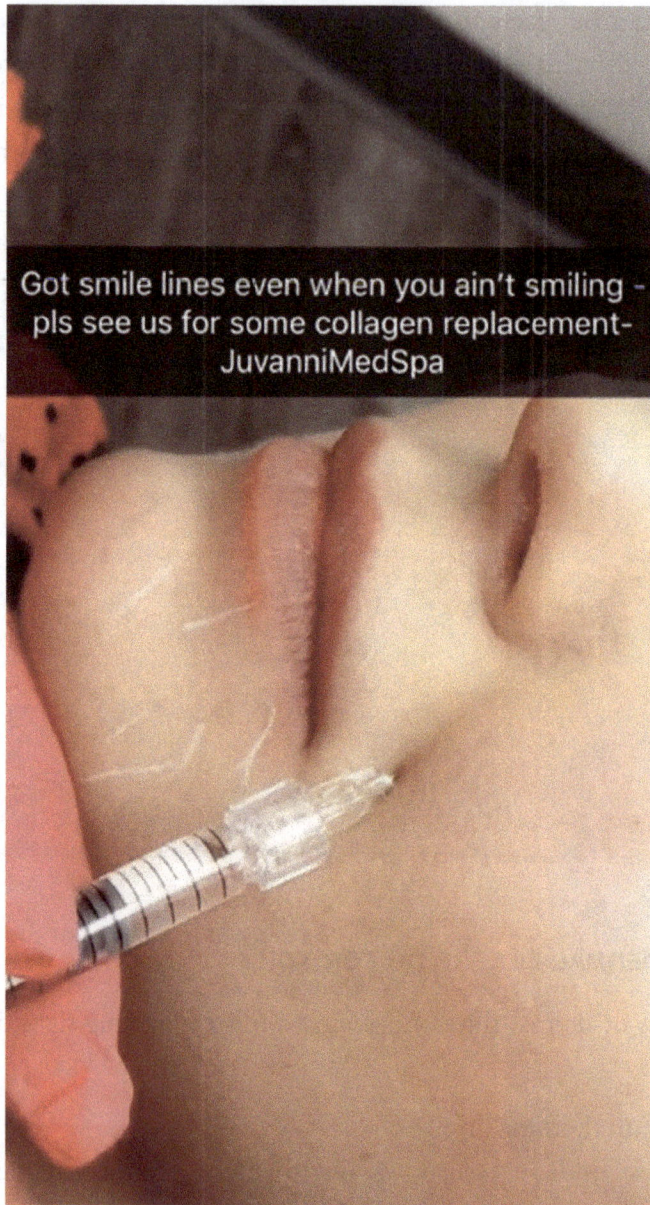

Got smile lines even when you ain't smiling - pls see us for some collagen replacement- JuvanniMedSpa

DERMAL FILLERS: RISKS AND CONSIDERATIONS

Dermal fillers are generally considered safe, but side effects are possible. The side effects are usually injector dependent, and that's why selecting your injector carefully is important. The most common problems are:

- Skin rash or itching.
- Redness, bruising, or swelling.
- Undesirable results, such as asymmetry, lumps, or overcorrection of wrinkles.

- Skin damage that causes a wound, infection, or scarring.
- Being able to feel the filler under the skin (for a few weeks after injection).
- Blindness, if filler is injected in an artery that is close to the blood supply of the eye (extremely rare).
- Death of skin cells due to loss of blood flow to the area. This is called intravascular necrosis, and if this happens, some of the hyaluronic acid fillers can be easily melted. But if the injector has placed the kind of fillers that can't be melted, you are in trouble. Go to the nearest ER with a very good plastic surgeon.

These rare cases are as uncommon as the odds of getting in a car wreck that leads to horrible physical damage. However, given that some of these complications are severe, you should choose an experienced and reputable doctor with a verifiable record of success if you choose to use dermal fillers.

What to do before and after cosmetic injections

BEFORE FILLER

@lipfillerscollective

AVOID	AVOID	DON'T
blood thinning tablets 2 weeks before	alcohol 48 hours before	exercise 24 hours before

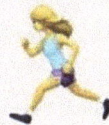

2/2

AFTER FILLER

@lipfillerscollective

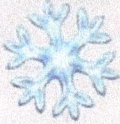

DO
ice for 24-48 hours after

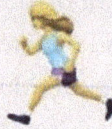

DON'T
exercise 24 hours after

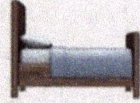

DON'T
lie down, keep elevated

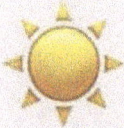

AVOID
sun exposure

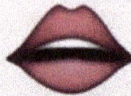

DON'T
rub or massage your lips

DO
take herbal supplements like arnica or bromelain

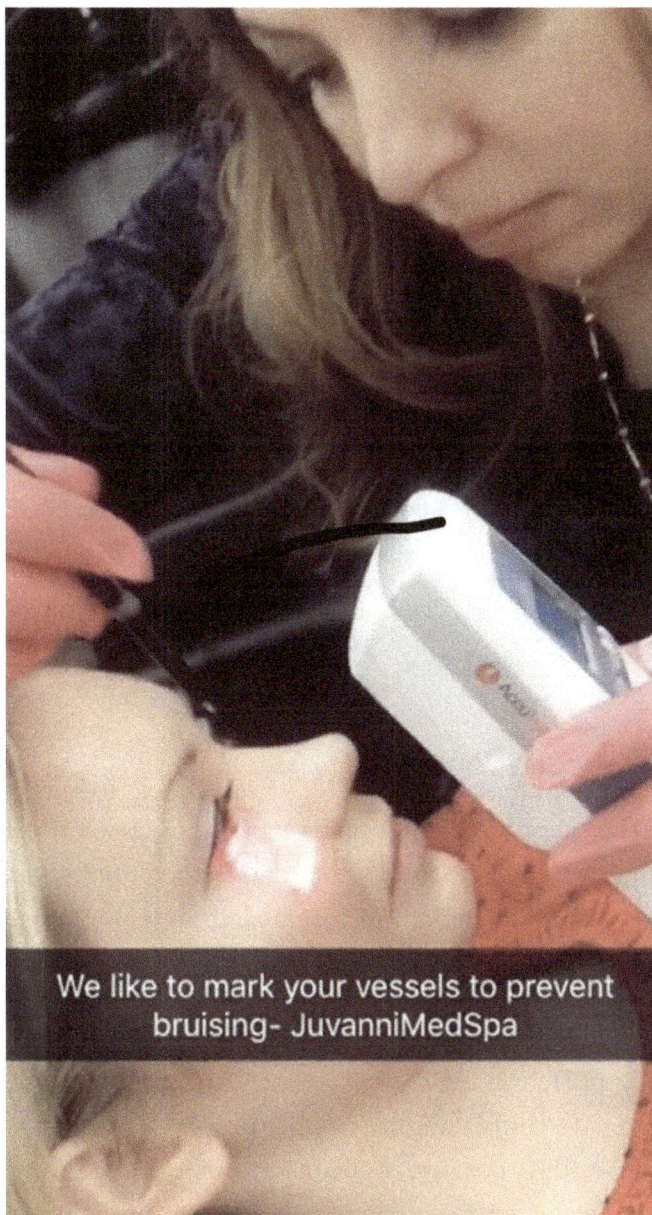

We like to mark your vessels to prevent bruising- JuvanniMedSpa

AccuVein (an ultrasound to detect blood vessels under the skin) is a useful tool used before injecting dermal fillers. It helps in mapping blood vessels before injecting.

The cost of dermal filler treatments varies from one provider to another and depends on the procedure performed, the treatment area, and the quality of the dermal filler used. But the value of a beauty expert who is also an experienced and safe injector is immeasurable.

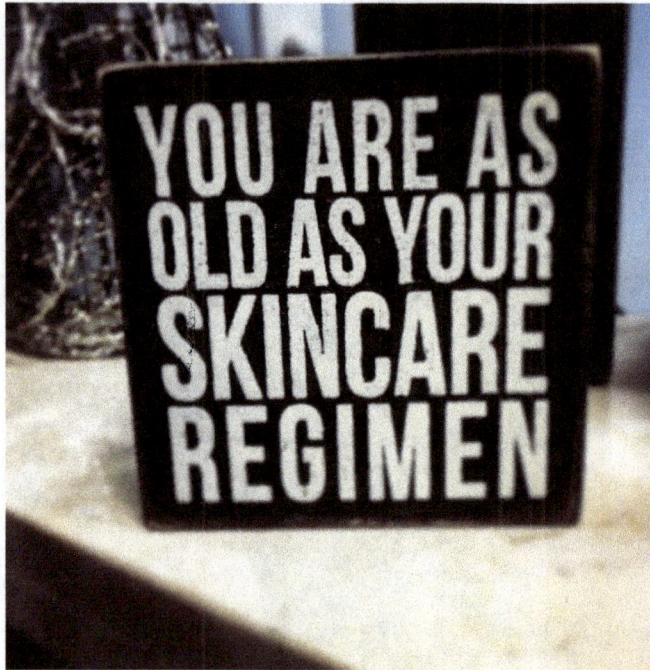

At what age should you start?

The answer to this question depends on a variety of factors. Your skin age and condition reflect your DNA, your environment, the food, alcohol, pollution, and smoke that you put in your body, and the amount of mental and physical stress you endure on a daily basis.

Have I injected young adults in their early 20s? Yes, I have. I always congratulate young people for being proactive about their wellness rather than passively waiting until they start looking old. Millennials are my favorite people and my target population to train about wellness. Health is not just about the absence of disease, and millennials seems to understand this. They know that even though their lives are going to be more chaotic, they will live longer than previous generations. So, they want to live well. However, they must learn to decipher between the good, the bad, and the stupid advances in modern aesthetics. They must also learn to think outside the box—because in real life, there is no box.

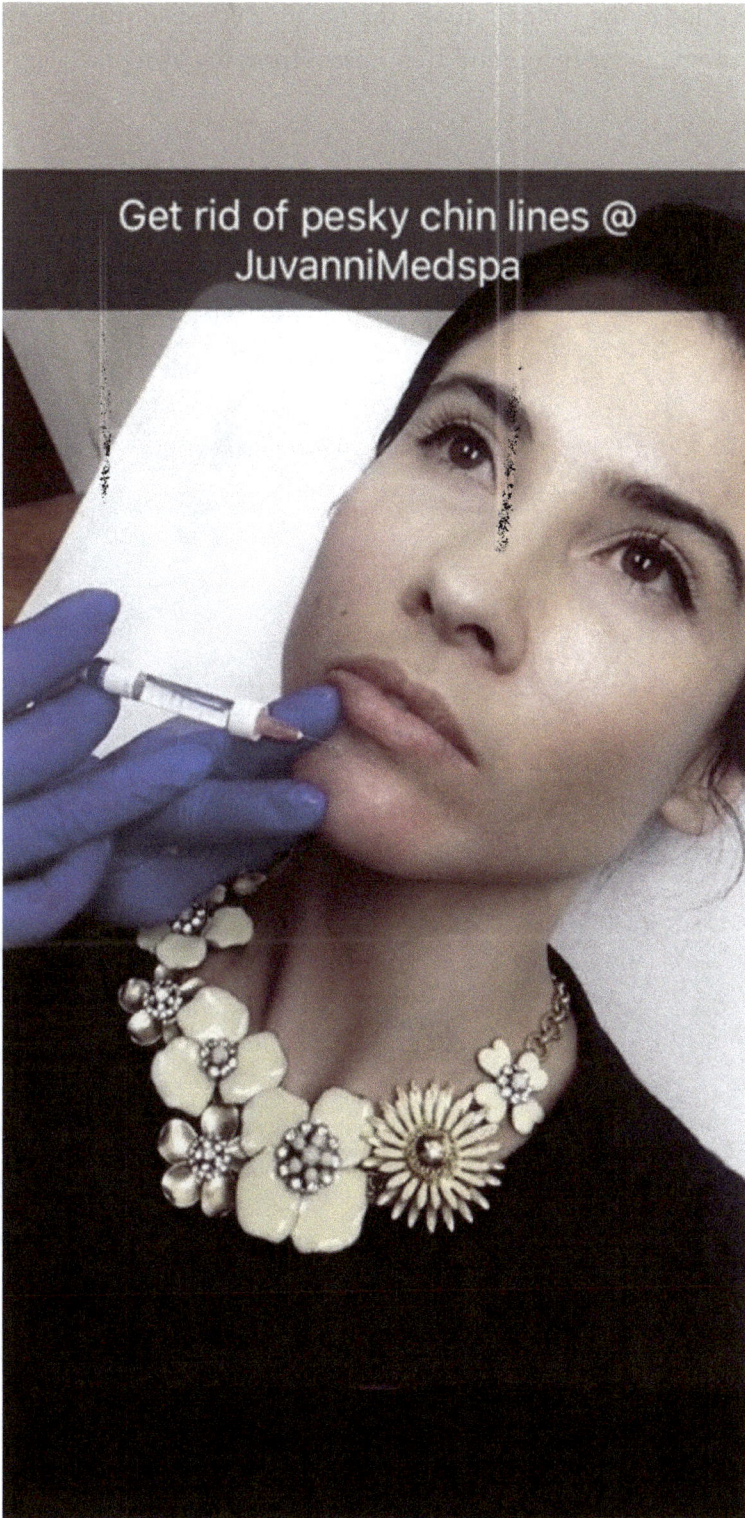

Get rid of pesky chin lines @ JuvanniMedspa

To help you judge for yourself about the possible effects of using dermal fillers, here's a gallery of representative before and after images from my own practice:

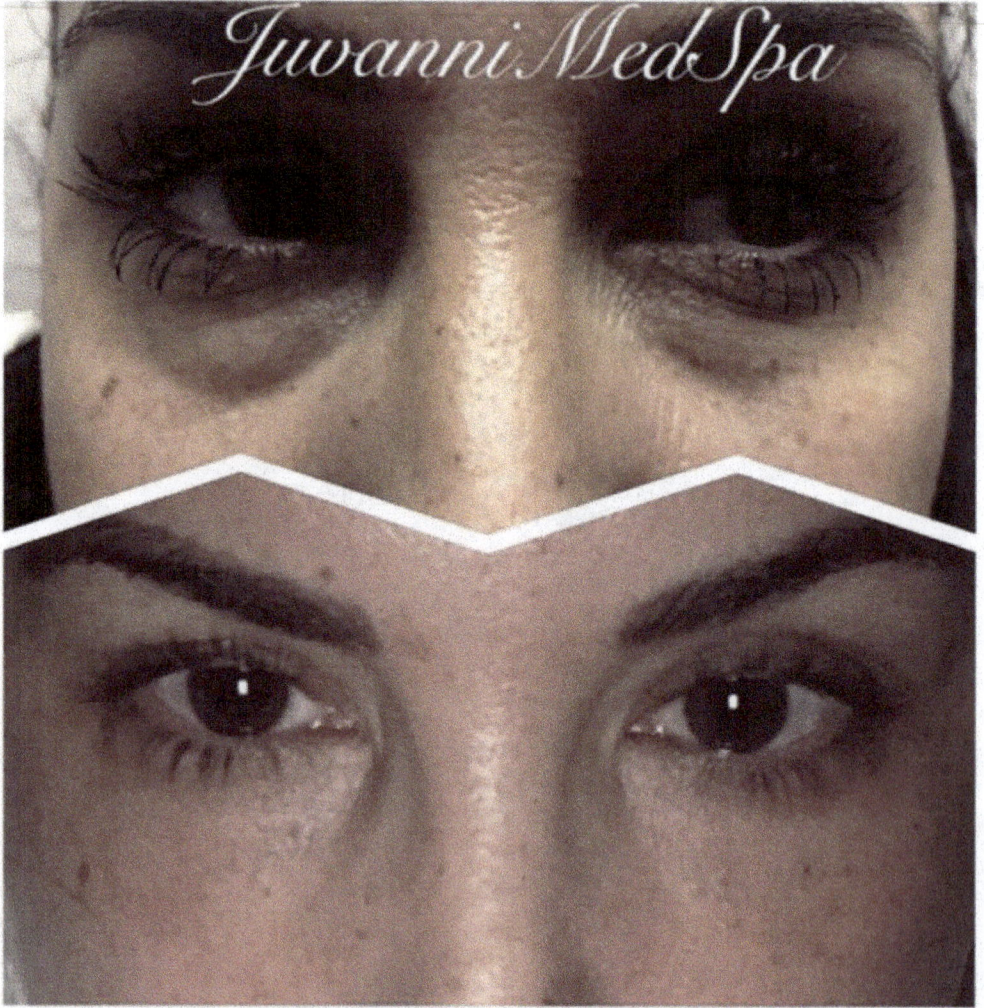

The Countless Tales of Befores and Afters (1)

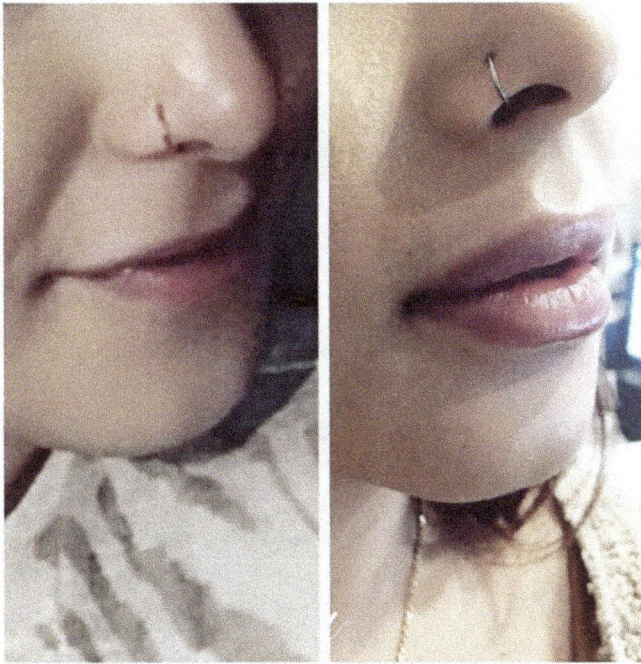

The Countless Tales of Befores and Afters (2)

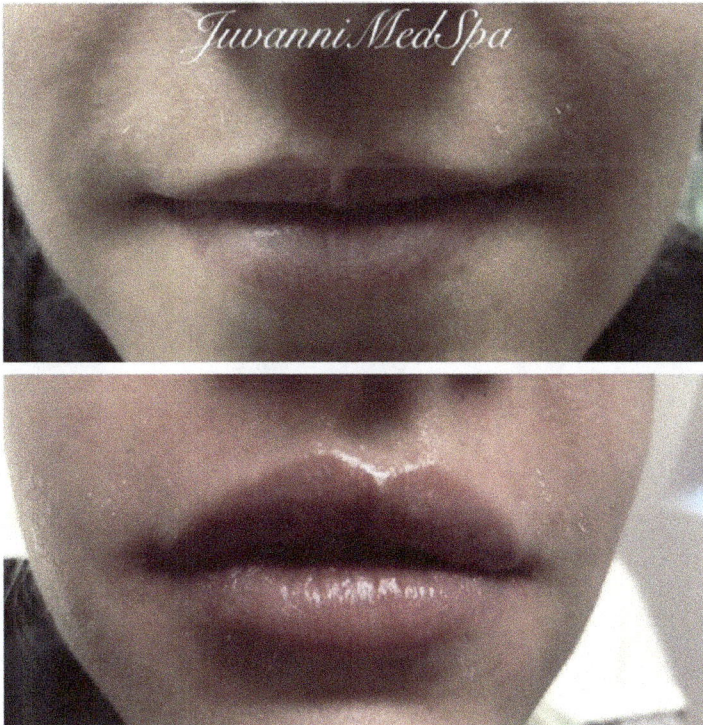

The Countless Tales of Befores and Afters (3)

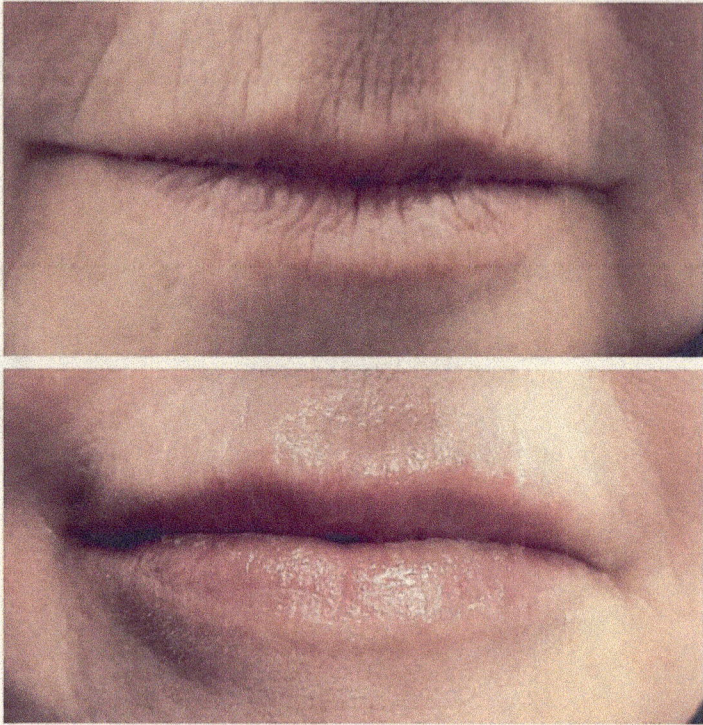

The Countless Tales of Befores and Afters (4)

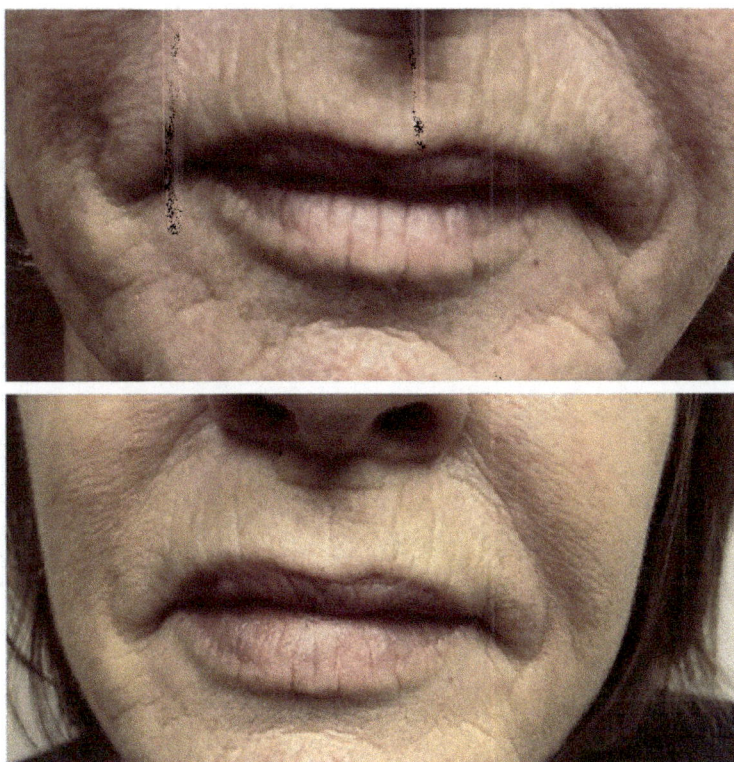

The Countless Tales of Befores and Afters (5)

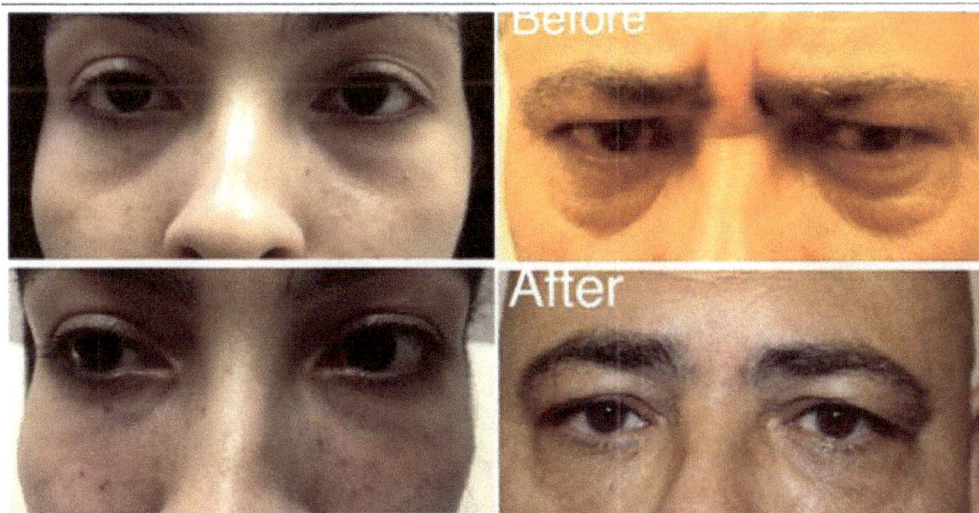

The Countless Tales of Befores and Afters (I'm losing count…)

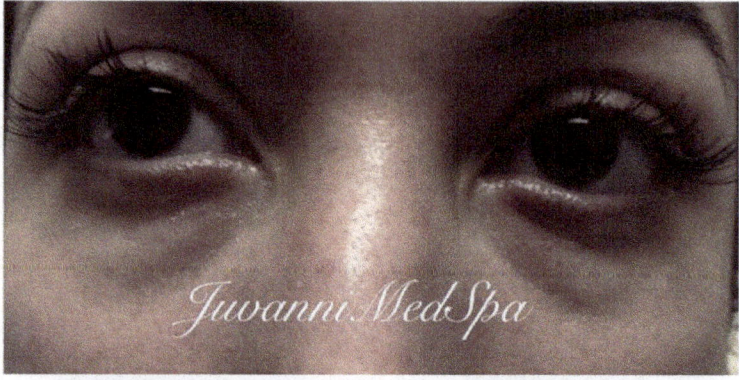

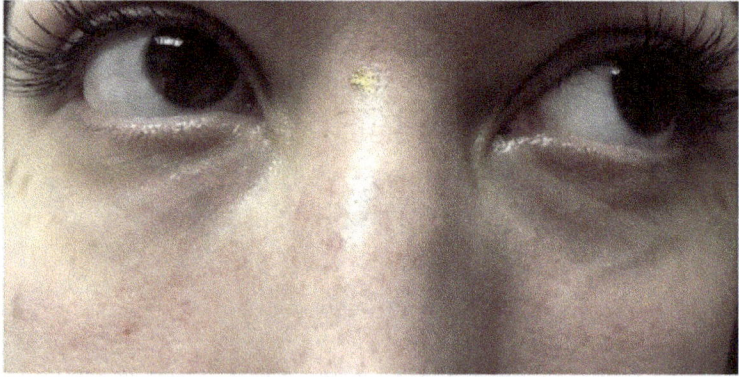

The Countless Tales of Befores and Afters (I lost count . . .)

Chapter 4

Allergan, I love you.
Allergan, I hate you.

When I came to America, I did part-time substitute teaching at a local high school. The kids would sometimes unite in hating or loving a teacher, bonding with each other over their shared love or disdain for the next 45 minutes of class. Some kids would try to weasel their way onto my good side, becoming proverbial teacher's pets. Others would be backbenchers like I was, keeping their heads down and never getting in any trouble. In Botox-Land and Fillerville, Allergan is the teacher, and there are some other small companies who, like the teacher's pet, just go whatever direction Allergan establishes for them.

Since Allergan is the teacher of Botox-Land, he is very important. Almost all aesthetic providers want him to be better than what he is now. Allergan has expanded very rapidly, and the prices of its cosmetic products are skyrocketing with regular yearly increases. Very soon, only the very wealthy will be able to afford these products. Allergan won't stop and rethink its market strategy for anti-aging, but people and governments must.

Is the world ready to be divided into the rich people who always look beautiful and young at any age, and the poor who look pretty for only five or ten years?

A slightly more futuristic version of this worry animates Yuval Noah Harari's *Homo Deus*, where he envisions a near future in which differential access to prenatal genetic engineering differentiates human beings into two broad and readily apparent strata, the unmodified with various imperfections and a normal range of IQs, heights, athletic abilities, physical appearances, etc.; and the modified, perfect specimens of humanity. At a more superficial level, I am concerned this dystopian future is rapidly materializing in the present in part thanks to aesthetic and anti-aging medicine and companies like Allergan.[16]

---

[16] Harari, *Homo Deus: A Brief History of Tomorrow*, (New York: Harper, 2017).

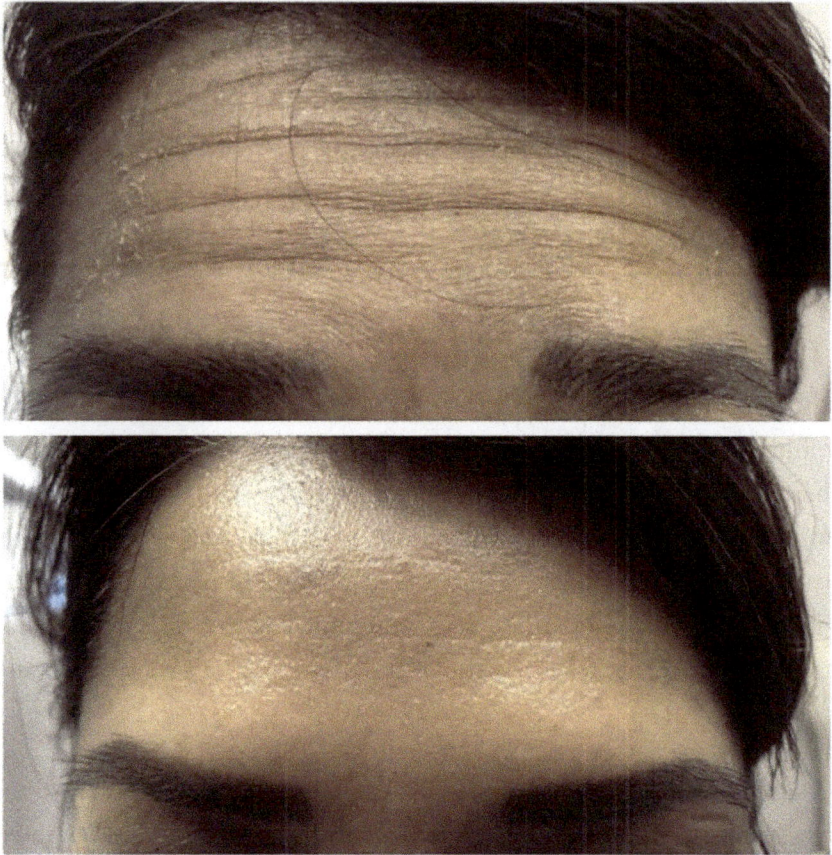

Forehead wrinkles before and after Botox

Allergan owns Botox and recently acquired CoolSculpting by Zeltiq. I joke with my clients all the time that I would have made more money buying stock in Zeltiq and Allergan (I currently own no stock in either company) instead of their products. But then I remember the famous line I heard somewhere: "We have to love the shit sandwich we chose to eat." I am totally passionate about these treatments and how they help ordinary people's lives and keep providing them at reasonable prices. This is a medication that people need every three months as they enter their 40s. They will typically use approximately 40 to 60 units each time, so providing reasonable prices is important to making these treatments accessible.

Her: he's probably thinking about other girls

Him: when will she stop spending so much money on filler...

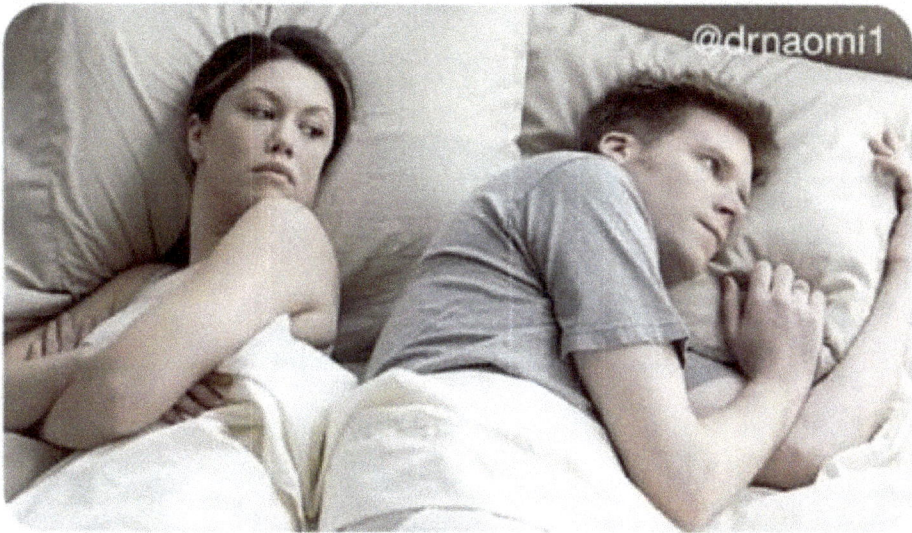

Life is difficult, and that's before pharmaceutical companies make it expensive.

The cost of Botox and other similar products is roughly six or seven dollars per unit for a business. If you are a large buyer, you can perhaps get a better deal at five or six dollars per unit, which you sell at 15 dollars to make a profit. My clients like the price to be stabilized at 10 to 12 dollars per unit. Is it possible? It is very difficult to price Botox at that rate without having to do a lot of treatments. Instead, medical practices join like-minded wellness providers to form groups and demand lower prices. Since there are competing companies, cheaper prices can be negotiated. Doctors should become part of this negotiation.

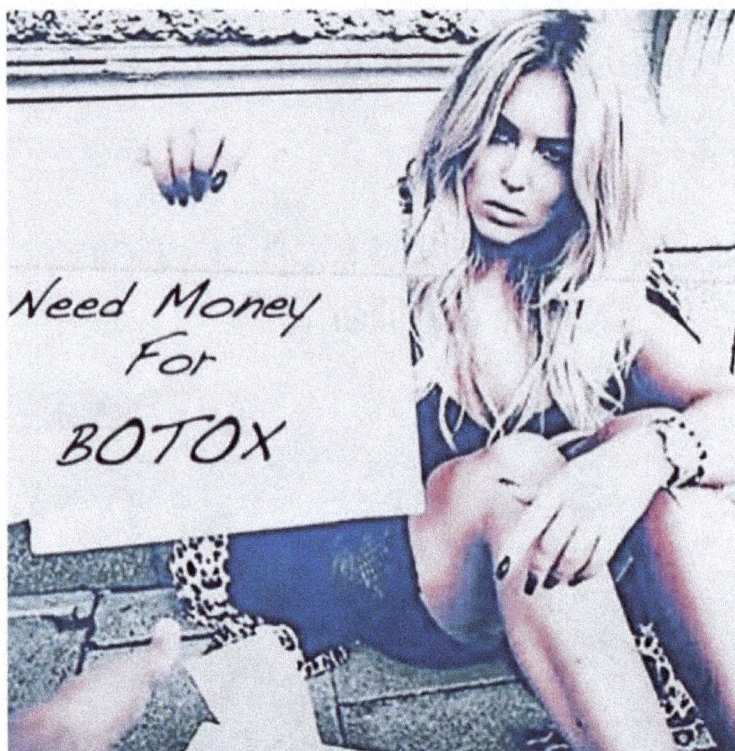

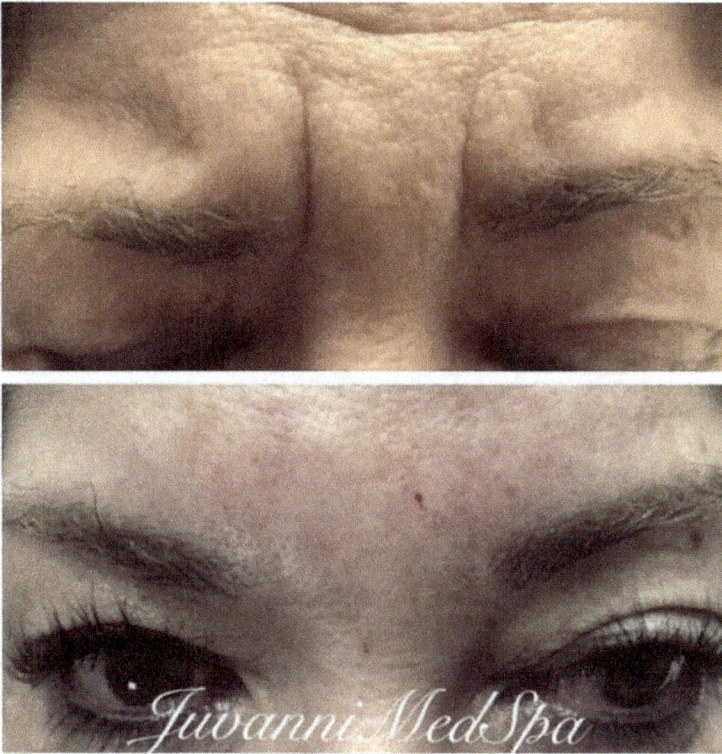

Frown lines before and after Botox and dermal filler

Other products similar to Botox include:

- **Xeomin** is Merz's answer to Botox and can be more affordable. If you get Xeomin at 12 dollars per unit, be happy. Its dosing is similar to Botox but does not last quite as long. Xeomin is a safer product than Botox for people with a history of cancer or a transplant. I especially love it because it's the first toxin I ever injected in someone else.

- **Dysport** is produced by Galderma and is the younger, stronger, and longer-lasting rival of Botox.

- **Jeuveau** is the new kid on the block. I offer it in my practice and find it to be comparable to Botox with a slightly better price point.

- **Revance** is an upcoming attraction and probably longer lasting than Botox. (It is supposed to last twice as long.) I am sure many clients will prefer something that lasts longer, but that could be problematic if you have a bad side effect.

Juvanni Med Spa
www.juvanni.com
(914)-368-6609

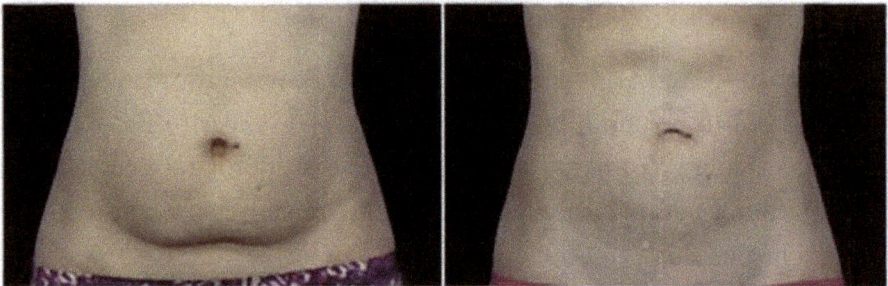

BEFORE   16 WEEKS AFTER

Abdominal fat before and after CoolSculpting (also owned by Allergan)

I think the only way any of the companies can ever stand out and claim market share from Botox and Allergan is if they get their product accepted by health insurance for routine anti-aging. Alternatively, costs will come down if and when a form of Botox is developed that can be administered topically. Personally, I am waiting for a topical Botox that is covered by health insurance.

Chapter 5

Food for Thought

First of All, What is Food, and Why is it Getting Harder to Find?

Food is the essence of our being. We are not like plants, which have this magnificent gift of converting sunlight, air, and water into food through photosynthesis. We have to get our food from other sources. Don't get me wrong—I like being human, but getting food from my environment can be problematic these days. The food environment in the United States and much of the rest of the world has been radically transformed over the past few decades to the point that most food is so unhealthy it's practically toxic. Furthermore, the food industry has an increasingly advanced understanding of how our brains work. As a result, they are able to produce "engineered food" to manipulate our brain chemistry (specifically the food-reward circuitry of the limbic system). Instead of focusing on your health, the food industrial complex's focus is on maximizing consumption, which maximizes their profits. Being healthy in the 21st century and maintaining health and vitality thus requires being thoughtful and critical about what one eats.

Michael Pollan, a prolific and illuminating writer about food (who also has numerous talks and podcasts available on the web) repeatedly comes back to the same principle: you are what you eat. Your health, weight gain, sustained weight loss, long-term disease susceptibility, complexion—everything depends squarely upon what you eat.

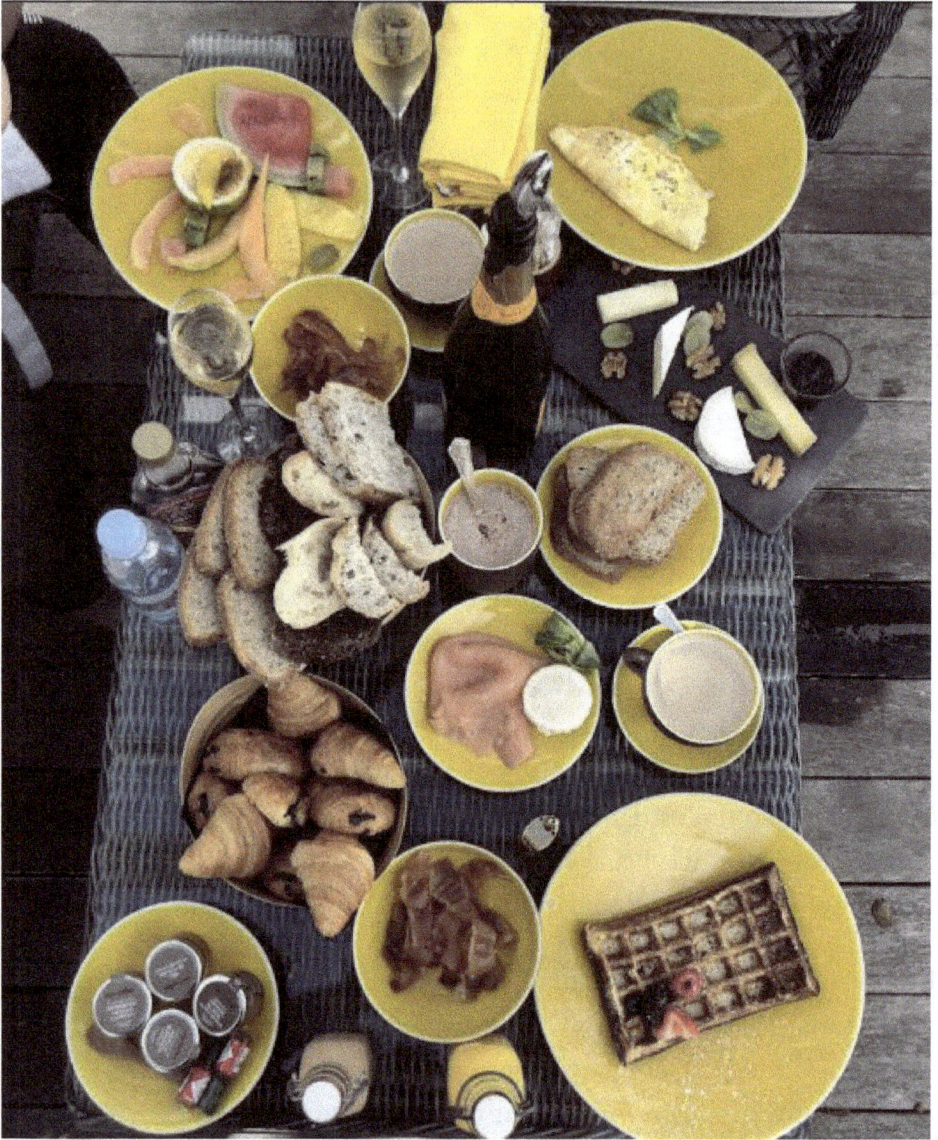

At the end of the first chapter, I shared an automobile metaphor I often tell my patients: If you want to transform your Honda into a Mercedes, you can't concentrate on the outer shell alone. You also need to upgrade the engine. The way we change our engines to become healthier, more attractive, thriving people is by eating well and exercising regularly. From an early age, we face considerable societal influences and temptations that could inhibit our health and positive body image. Although there may be an abundance of seemingly delicious food, to be healthy we have to learn to identify and resist the temptation of highly processed and addictive "food" products and eat real food instead.

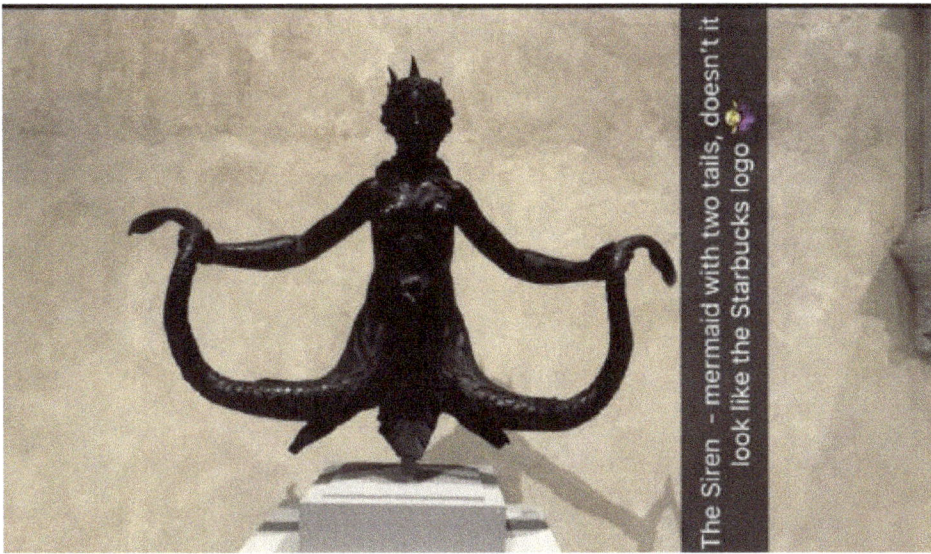

The Siren – mermaid with two tails, doesn't it look like the Starbucks logo

The nation of burgers has become the nation of Starbucks, but at least Starbucks had the subtle honesty to hide their business model in plain sight in their logo featuring the siren, the mythological personification of destructive temptation.

The main culprit here is the industrial food production system that gets you addicted to bad food for the sake of profits. This system is relatively new—it has its origins in post–World War II developments in fertilizers, pesticides, and technology, and really took hold only in the past four decades. To give credit where it is due, these revolutions in food production techniques and technology make it possible to feed a much larger population around the world and for most Americans to spend less than half what they spent on food just a couple of generations ago. But the other side of this coin is that United States agribusiness produces roughly 4,000 calories per person per day, practically double what most of us need. The majority of these calories are in the form of products like corn and soy, which cannot even be ingested by humans without being highly processed (hence corn syrup and soy oil), or meat that is loaded with antibiotics and steroids instead of nutrients.

Furthermore, the U.S. federal government actually subsidizes the overproduction of unhealthy food, and it appears to be more interested in preventing people from learning how bad certain foods are (hence the cryptic labeling discussed below) rather teaching people how to eat well. In short, there is an incredibly powerful, trillion-dollar-a-year industry working against us.

yuval_noah_harari ✓   ···

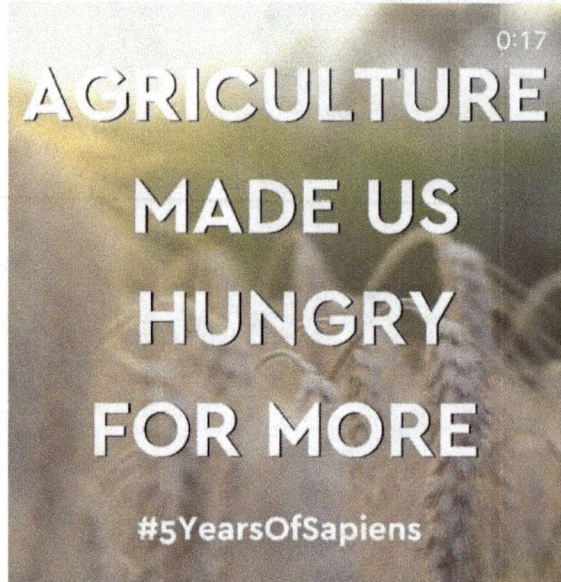

0:17

AGRICULTURE MADE US HUNGRY FOR MORE

#5YearsOfSapiens

♡ ○ ◁   🔖

12,860 views

yuval_noah_harari "The Agricultural Revolution certainly enlarged the sum total of food at the disposal of humankind, but the extra... more

Choosing the right food is the key to living and thriving in the matrix of our existence. But what is the right food? The media keeps us confused and lures us with myths—"This food will rid you of all our toxins." "Meet the new superfood!" We have food pundits ready to blast each other about which is the magic food and which is the evil culprit. There are multiple studies published each year, often funded by the industry that stands to benefit if their results are accepted, and they often contain conflicting information, leading to even more confusion. So, what food is the right food?

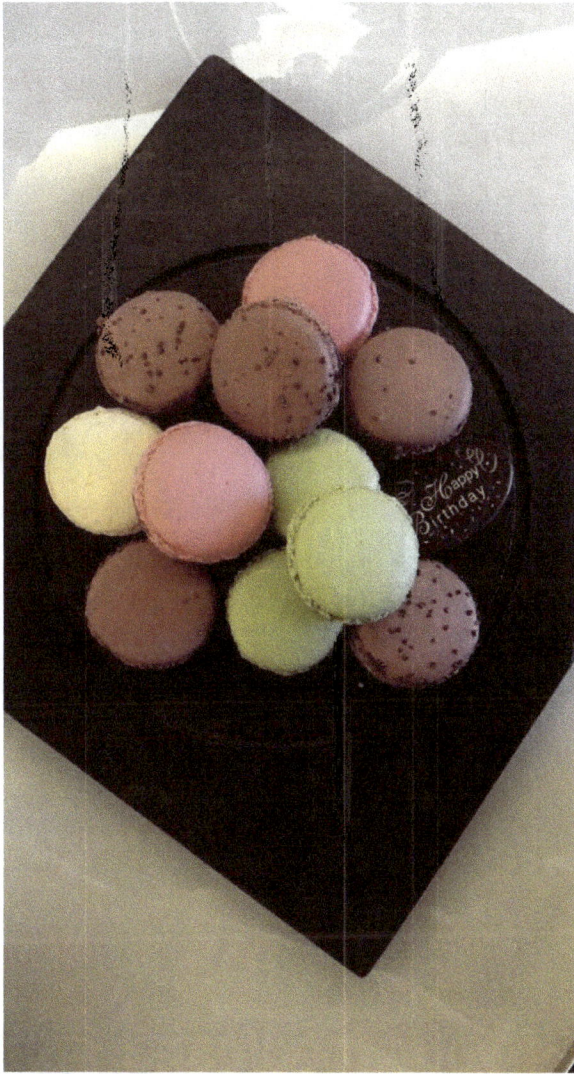

Let's start with the more basic question: What exactly *is* food? Mark Bittman, *New York Times* food columnist and author of a bookshelf full of great cookbooks, says it best. He emphasizes healthy, ethical approaches to food for the 21st century and points out that, if you start with a straightforward definition of food—that it's a nutritious substance that people eat or drink in order to maintain health and growth—then around 60% of the edible offerings at your average grocery store are not food. Instead, most of what is sold as food in the U.S. and many other advanced economies today is so highly processed and loaded with sugars, fats, preservatives, and additives that a diet that regularly features these items does little to sustain our health and vitality. By some estimates, as much as 75% of healthcare expenses in the U.S. go to fight preventable chronic diseases linked to diet!

"Metabolic syndrome" is a term coined by Robert Lustig, an endocrinologist and leading public health doctor at the University of California, San Francisco Medical School. It refers to a family of diseases (obesity, diabetes, heart disease, stroke, cancer, and perhaps dementia) that we address without tackling the root cause—our dysfunctional food production and marketing system. The outcome is bankrupting the American healthcare system.[17]

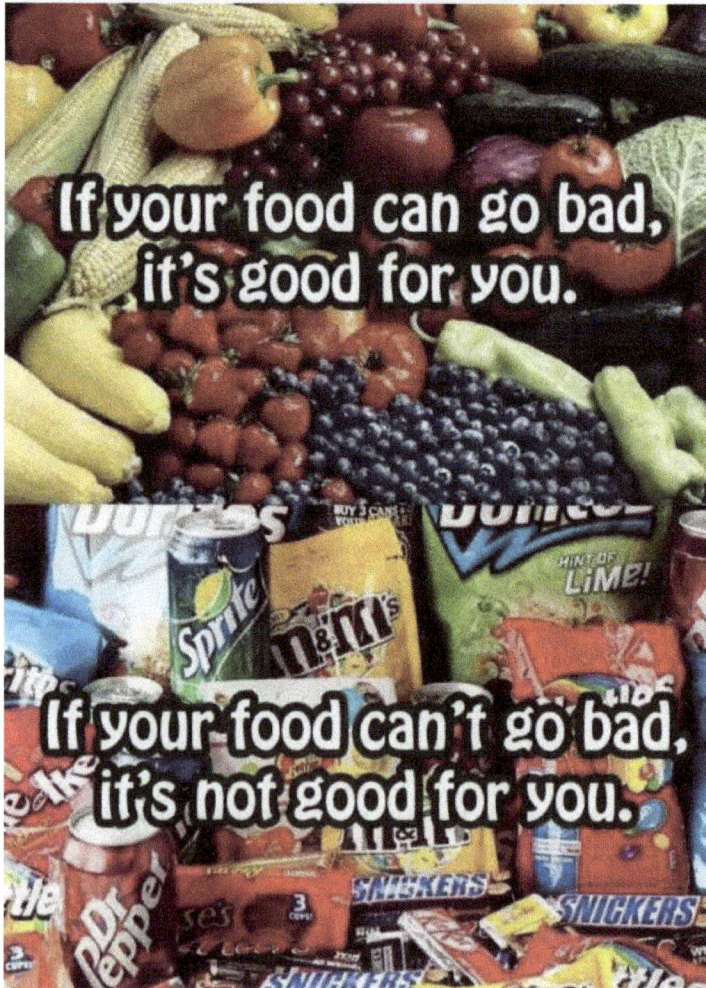

For the sake of our kids, our fellow citizens, and the planet, we should support public policy to better regulate and tax the industrial food production system and to create greater transparency and awareness about the connection between bad food, diet, obesity, and disease. I believe we need to realize that eating is the new smoking and demand that

---

[17] See Lustig, *The Hacking the American Mind*, op. cit.

our governments take steps to address the epidemic of bad food consumption, just as they did to address the public health concerns surrounding the tobacco industry.

But I'm not holding my breath for government action in the current political climate, so in addition we must make *ourselves* healthier and the environment more sustainable by eating better. The place to start is recognizing that much of what is sold in grocery stores and restaurants today isn't really food. It's not nourishing and sustaining us, just making us fat and sick—leading to the spread of disease both directly (what we eat leads to diabetes, heart disease, etc.) and indirectly (when animals are fed in lots and pumped full of hormones and steroids, we create the perfect petri dish for growing antibiotic-resistant superbugs). Furthermore, the existing system is cruel to animals, bad for the soil, and ultimately unsustainable. So the first and most important rule of an anti-aging diet is to eat real food!

EDUCATING YOURSELF ABOUT FOOD

As a single mother working six days a week for unpredictably long hours, I found that grocery shopping on days off and cooking every day was simply not sustainable. So I hired a cook to prepare meals for my daughter and me. But I was hardly able to eat these homemade meals. I was always at work and ate restaurant meals many days. Good restaurant food is wonderful as an occasional treat but not great on a regular basis. It is prepared to be so delicious that you keep wanting to eat more. But eating more can be harmful.

In Pakistan, I used to eat home-cooked meals made by either my mom or the chefs that my parents would keep to attend to the kitchen. The food was usually simple: lentils, lots of veggies, sometimes dessert, and (once or twice a week) meat. When I came to America, my husband's diet was like nothing I had ever experienced. Food from all over the world was available in almost every town. But who cares about that when McDonald's tastes so good? And oh my God, check out the potato wedges from KFC—and did you taste the new hard taco at Taco Bell . . . ?

I was a size two when I came to the U.S., and I am not telling *anyone* my current size. I have had a whole bunch of CoolSculpting done to combat my stress-relieving habits (like overeating bad food). *You can't just exercise (or CoolSculpt) your way out of a bad diet!*

That lesson took me a couple decades to learn, and adhering to it remains a daily challenge for me. *Food addiction is perhaps as bad as alcohol or cigarette addiction,* and at the neurological level they are all quite similar. Having battled all three at different points in my life, I can say that food is the trickier battle to fight—we have to eat to survive. If you've become addicted or habituated to bad food, you can't just go cold turkey—you have to retrain yourself to enjoy good food, which means that you need to be able to tell the difference between healthy, nutritious sources of sustenance and the crap that the food industrial complex markets as food.

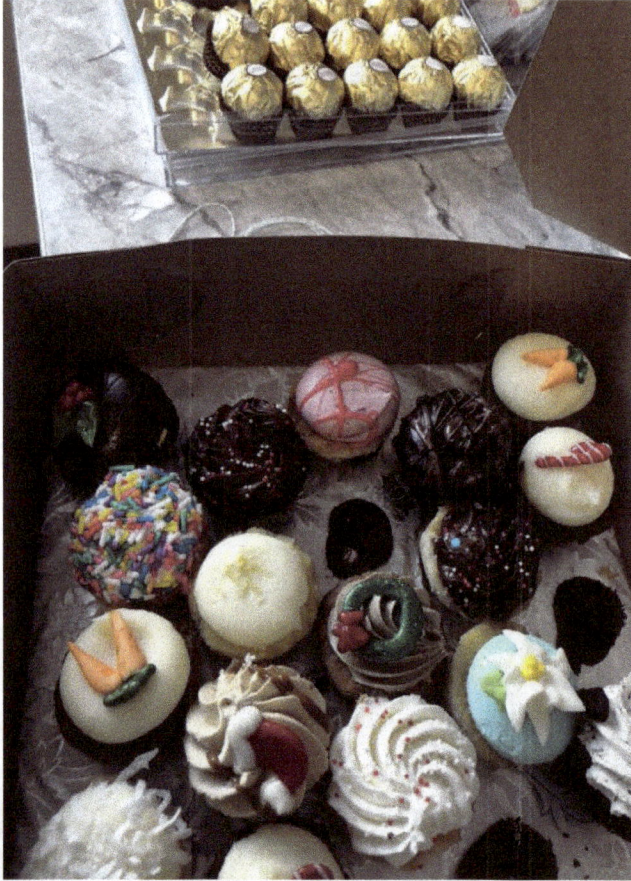

Christmas treats from clients at the office—thanks, no thanks!

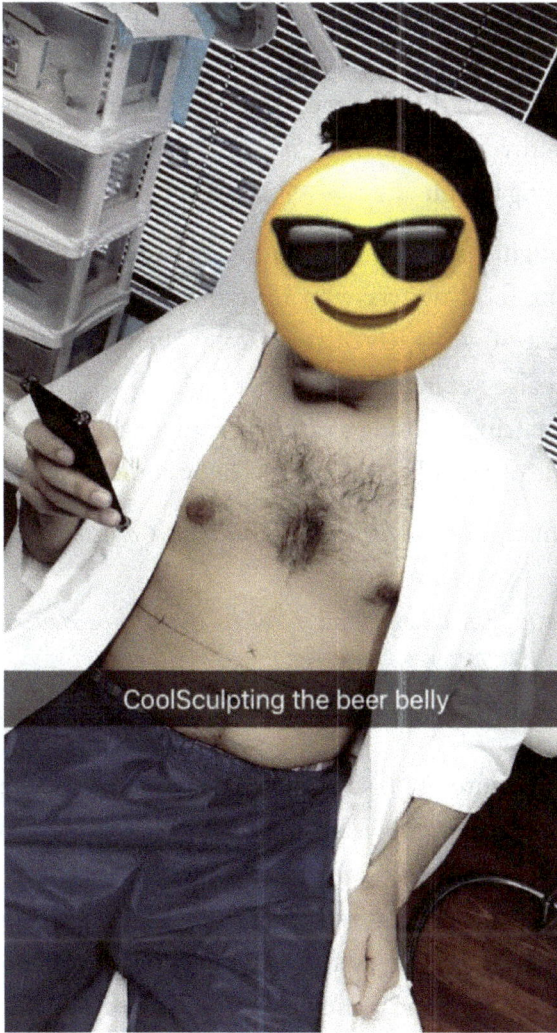

CoolSculpting the beer belly

In the following chapter, I will discuss diets and will have plenty to say about what has worked for me and many of my patients. But I want to start with more basic advice on food and nutrition. If you develop the habit of eating healthy on a regular basis, you will stop craving unhealthy food, maybe even be disgusted by it once you recognize what's in it and see what it's doing to you.

There is nothing original in what I'm about to summarize here—it's based on the work of a group of brilliant food writers who have documented how transformations in food systems over the last 50 years have dramatically changed diets and health. These are not only important but also fascinating, illuminating, and well-written works, so next time you are going on a plane trip, choosing a vacation read, or thinking about delving into the next diet fad, pick up one of the following books. They could change your life.

- Mark Bittman, *Food Matters: A Guide to Conscious Eating with More Than 75 Recipes*
- Robert Lustig, *Fat Chance* and *The Hacking of the American Mind*
- Marion Nestle, *What to Eat*
- Michael Pollan, *The Omnivore's Dilemma* and *Food Rules: An Eater's Manual*

Without going too far into the historical details (you can get these from any of the books just mentioned), over the last 50 years, food systems in much of the developed world have transitioned away from traditional agriculture based on a rotation of diverse crops, relatively small-scale farming, pasture raising, and a mainly self-sustaining nutrient cycle. In its place, we have a monoculture system built on single crops dominated by corn and soy, petroleum-based fertilizers and pesticides, and animals raised in feedlots. This is an environmental nightmare, contributing to global warming and unsustainable food consumption habits. (As I write these words, the Amazon rainforest is on fire to provide space to raise cattle and soy.) If the Chinese replicate the American diet, we will need 2.3 Earths to feed them and us together—never mind the other 6 billion humans on earth!

It's also a health disaster. The new agribusiness farming system produces much more industrial raw materials than food—forms of soy and corn that need to be chemically processed in order to be turned into food (e.g., high fructose corn syrup or soy protein and oil) or fed to animals. As a result of these changes, *the average American now eats around 40 pounds of high fructose corn syrup in a year (down from 63 pounds per year 20 years ago), and 10% of calories in the average American diet comes from soy oil.*

As this industry has pushed more poor-quality calories into the food system, an increasingly high proportion of the calories we consume comes from added sugars or saturated fats, and from meat and refined carbohydrates. Americans consequently consume somewhere between 250 and 500 more calories per person per day than they were eating just 40 years ago, and weigh almost 20 pounds more than they did in 1980. This is the overweight and obesity epidemic, and it is associated with many other diseases and co-morbidities.

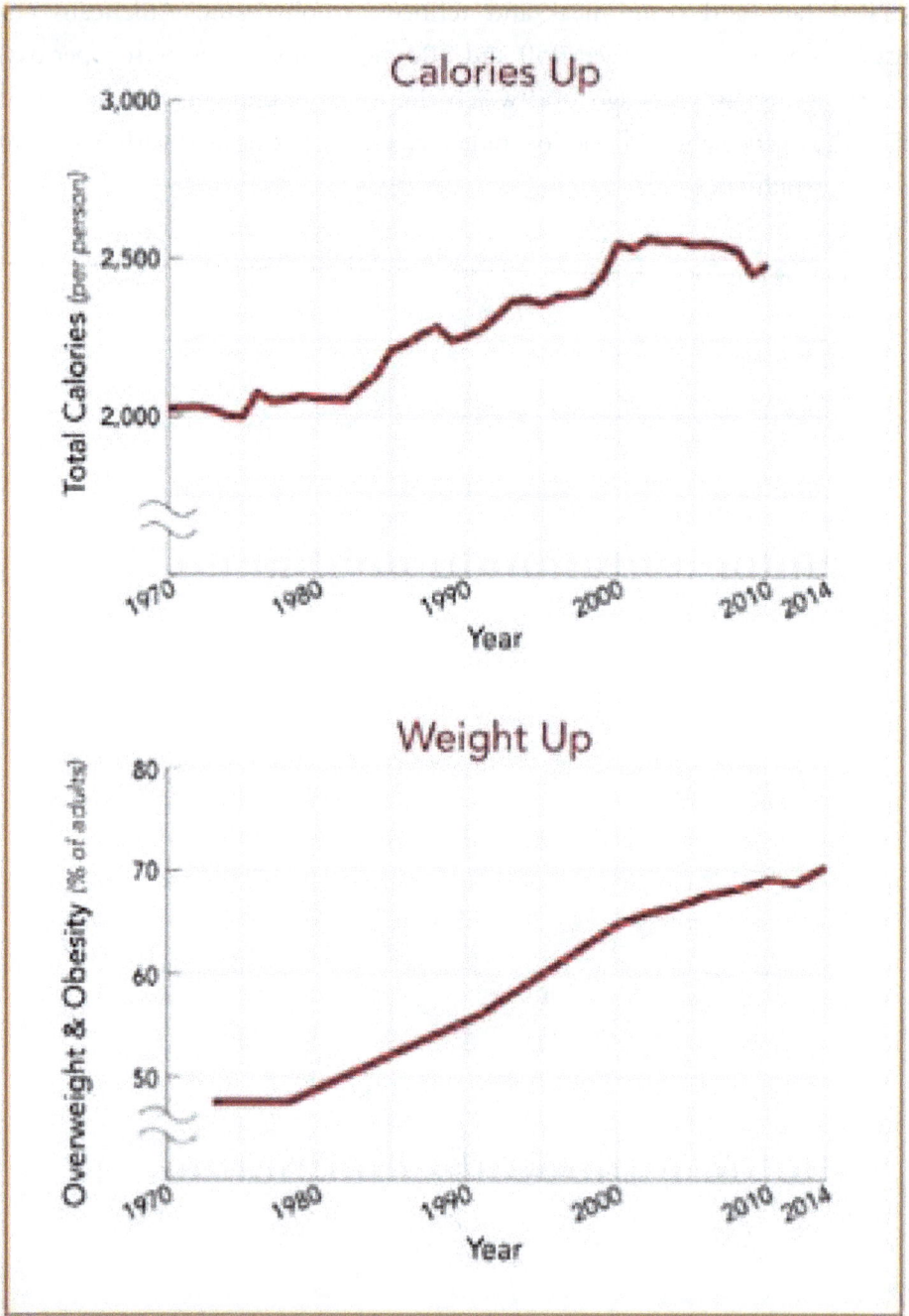

Diagram 1: The Great Calorie Push: Calories in the food supply started climbing around 1980, and so did the percentage of adults who are overweight or obese.[18]

---

[18] Diagram source: NAH Editorial Staff, "A leading researcher explains the obesity epidemic," *Nutrition Action Healthletter*, August 1, 2018, (https://www.nutritionaction.com/daily/diet-and-weight-loss/a-leading-researcher-explains-the-obesity-epidemic/_), (Site visiting September 2, 2019).

It all comes down to this: We are what we eat, and most of us eat way too much crap. In many respects, this is not our fault. Our government encouraged the transformation of our food system, and beginning in the 1970s, it subsidized the overproduction of unhealthy foods. Instead of making it easy for us to figure out what's healthy and what's not, the FDA is in the pocket of the industries it "regulates" and helps camouflage what's in our food and how bad it is for us. And the media does too little to assist us here as well. Often food-related research is funded by the very industry that produces the substances being studied, producing results the industry wants us to see.[19] Far too often the "attention merchants" in the media broadcast this manipulation because they know a sensational headline ("Red Meat Isn't So Bad for You After All") will keep your eyes on their page or site.

So what can you do? Become an educated consumer, which means cultivating a healthy skepticism about many of the claims made in commercials, restaurants, and the popular press about the health benefits of various "food" products. Since Upton Sinclair published *The Jungle* in 1906 to expose the unsanitary conditions in the meatpacking industry, many Americans have been at least somewhat aware of a lack of transparency in the food industry. It's hard to regulate or intelligently consume from an industry you don't understand. So, *caveat emptor* ("buyer beware"). Arm yourself to penetrate the deception and gain the knowledge you need to eat well. The bad news is that there aren't easy shortcuts to the knowledge you need—at some point, you will need to pick up one or more of the books listed above, and then stay up to speed with recent developments.[20] The good news is that, if you're like me (dyslexic and more partial to podcasts and social media than long books), you may be pleasantly surprised with how readable and interesting these works are. One thing I can say for sure: You will be on the path to a more thoughtful, critical, educated, and healthy approach to food and eating if you take the time to read at least one of these books.

A CRASH COURSE IN FOOD EDUCATION

Since you're reading this book now, one thing I can do is to give you a quick crash course in food education. This is not a substitute for the systematic books listed above, but at least it's a start. As mentioned at the end of the first section of this chapter, the first and most

---

[19] Bonnie Liebman, "Industry-funded Research Feeds the Confusion," *Nutrition Action Healthletter*, September 2019, p p.30ff.

[20] One extremely helpful resource is *The Nutrition Action Healthletter*, a short digest of findings in recent nutrition research published ten times per year by the Center for Science in the Public Interest. (See: <https://cspinet.org/nutrition-action-healthletter>.)

important rule of the anti-aging diet is: eat real food! So what's real food? Here's a simple formula:

Eat what grows from the land and is available in the ocean, but definitely not anything that your grandmother didn't have when she was young.

Here are some tips to help you eat what your grandma ate:

1. *Eat real food.* Avoid ultra-processed foods. (This is really just another way of saying *eat real food*).
2. *Eat organic food* whenever available and affordable.
3. *Eat meat and dairy sparingly*, if you eat them at all, and only from pasture-raised animals.
4. *Cook your own food.* (Taking it out of a box or freezer bag doesn't count.)
5. Buy from local farms when you can.

Let me take each of these points in turn, starting with...

Rule 1: Eat Real Food

An international research consortium of food scientists and nutritionists recently devised the NOVA food classification system, which sorts food into four categories based on how the food is produced and processed.[21] This approach is extremely helpful in determining how to eat real, healthy food.

NOVA Group 1 consists of unprocessed or minimally processed foods. NOVA scientists recommend that you make the unprocessed foods from Group 1 the basis for your diet. Unprocessed foods can go from farm to plate, meaning they are in the same form when prepared for eating as when they were grown on a plant or cut from an animal. Group 1 foods may also be minimally processed, which means inedible or unwanted parts are removed, or they are dried, ground, boiled, pasteurized, frozen, squeezed for juice, etc. to preserve them or make them easier to store or transport. This is what I primarily mean by *food* and is what you should mainly eat. You should buy the building blocks of your meal in a form you can recognize, and then season and cook them yourself so that you know exactly what you're eating.

---

[21] For a more detailed summary of the NOVA Food Groups and Dietary Guidelines, see: Carlos A. Monteiro, et. al., "NOVA. The star shines bright," *World Nutrition*, Vol. 7, No. 1-3, January-March 2016, (<https://archive.wphna.org/wp-content/uploads/2016/01/WN-2016-7-1-3-28-38-Monteiro-Cannon-Levy-et-al-NOVA.pdf>) (site visited 8/31/19).

NOVA Group 2 contains processed culinary ingredients (i.e., food obtained directly from Group 1 foods by pressing, refining, grinding, milling, etc.—think spices). They are used to prepare, season, and cook Group 1 foods to make them into varied and enjoyable home-cooked dishes. They are rarely consumed in the absence of Group 1 foods. There is nothing wrong with Group 2, as long as you don't go overboard on the salt or sugar.

NOVA Group 3 is *processed food.* These are relatively simple products made by adding two or three Group 2 ingredients to Group 1 foods, like sugar, oil, salt, or other substances and have been processed in relatively simple ways, such as cooking or fermenting (in the case of cheese and bread) to preserve the food or make it taste or look better. Canned vegetables, fruits, and legumes, salted or sugared nuts and seeds, cured or smoked meats, cheeses and freshly made bread, and beer and wine all belong in Group 3. While you should avoid eating Group 3 foods frequently and certainly not make them the basis of your diet, they are fine as an occasional treat or a smaller portion of a recipe or meal.

NOVA Group 4 consists of ultra-processed food and drink *products*. Note that the doctors and scientists of NOVA are careful not to refer to this group as food, because it's not. This is the stuff to avoid. Let me quote what they say, because it's a little hard to express the definition of Group 4 in plain language:

These are industrial formulations typically with five or more and usually many ingredients. Such ingredients often include those also used in processed foods, such as sugar, oils, fats, salt, anti-oxidants, stabilizers, and preservatives. Ingredients only found in ultra-processed products include substances not commonly used in culinary preparations, and additives whose purpose is to imitate sensory qualities of group 1 foods or of culinary preparations of these foods, or to disguise undesirable sensory qualities of the final product. Group 1 foods are a small proportion of or are even absent from ultra-processed products. Substances only found in ultra-processed products include some directly extracted from foods, such as casein, lactose, whey, and gluten, and some derived from further processing of food constituents, such as hydrogenated or interesterified oils, hydrolyzed proteins, soy protein isolate, maltodextrin, invert sugar and high fructose corn syrup.[22]

Another telltale sign that the food product in question belongs to Group 4 is that it has added color or dyes.

---

[22] Monteiro et. al., "NOVA. The star shines bright," op. cite, p .33.

The NOVA nutritionists say the following about Group 4 'food' products:

The main purpose of industrial ultra-processing is to create products that are ready to eat, to drink or to heat, liable to replace both unprocessed or minimally processed foods . . . Common attributes of ultra-processed products are hyper-palatability, sophisticated and attractive packaging, multimedia and other aggressive marketing to children and adolescents, health claims, high profitability, and branding and ownership by transnational corporations. Examples of typical ultra-processed products are: carbonated drinks; sweet or savory packaged snacks [e.g., potato chips]; ice-cream, chocolate, candies (confectionery); mass-produced packaged breads and buns; margarines and spreads; cookies (biscuits), pastries, cakes, and cake mixes; breakfast 'cereals', 'cereal' and 'energy' bars; 'energy' drinks; milk drinks, 'fruit' yoghurts and 'fruit' drinks; . . . 'health' and 'slimming' products such as powdered or 'fortified' meal and dish substitutes; and many ready to heat products including pre-prepared pies and pasta and pizza dishes; poultry and fish 'nuggets' and 'sticks', sausages, burgers, hot dogs, and other reconstituted meat products, and powdered and packaged 'instant' soups, noodles and desserts.

So the NOVA doctors are saying that none of the above is food, and Mark Bittman observes that 60% of the edible products sold in the average American supermarket isn't food. 1 + 1 = 2, right?

What's an Ultra-Processed Diet?

Here are two sample menus from Kevin Hall's study pitting an ultra-processed diet against an unprocessed diet.

ULTRA-PROCESSED	UNPROCESSED
Breakfast	
Pancakes with margarine and syrup Turkey sausage Tater tots Apple juice	Oatmeal with blueberries and almonds 2% milk
Lunch	
Turkey sandwich with American cheese and mayo on white bread Baked potato chips Diet ginger ale	Entrée salad with grilled chicken breast, farro, apples, grapes, and lemon vinaigrette
Dinner	
Cheeseburger French fries and ketchup Diet ginger ale	Beef tender roast Couscous with lemon and garlic Green beans Side salad with honey vinaigrette
Snack	
Sweetened greek yogurt Canned peaches in heavy syrup	Carrots Black bean hummus

For more information: BMJ Open 2016, doi:10.1136/bmjopen-2015-009892.

Diagram 2: Real Food versus an Ultra-Processed Diet[23]

So the first rule is (to repeat) *eat only real food*, and the NOVA categories help us to understand what that means. Primarily eat unprocessed foods from Group 1, seasoned with the processed culinary ingredients from Group 2. Minimize your consumption of Group 3 processed foods, limiting them to occasional treats. And do your very best to avoid the ultra-processed foods of Group 4 like you would avoid the slow-acting but addictive poison they are.

---

[23] Diagram source: NAH Editorial Staff, "A leading researcher explains the obesity epidemic," *Nutrition Action Healthletter*, August 1, 2018, (https://www.nutritionaction.com/daily/diet-and-weight-loss/a-leading-researcher-explains-the-obesity-epidemic/_), (Site visited on September 2, 2019).

Processing usually makes food safer for human consumption, but the food loses valuable nutrients (like vitamins and minerals) and gains not-so-valuable nutrients (like salt, sugar and fat). While most of us intuitively get why minimally processed foods are healthier, it's eye-opening to see what happens to the nutrient profile (specifically, calories, sugar and sodium) of a food as it moves from farm to factory to fork.

REAL FOOD ← → PROCESSED FOOD

LEGEND

= 10 Calories   = 1 tsp Sugar   ● = 100 mg sodium   O = Less than 100 mg sodium

PEACH (150g)	CANNED PEACHES (150g)	PACKAGED PEACH PIE (150g)
1 INGREDIENT	4 INGREDIENTS	16 INGREDIENTS
55 Calories	80 Calories	335 Calories
3 ¼ tsp sugar	5 tsp sugar	
0mg Sodium	8mg Sodium	6 tsp sugar
		350mg Sodium

Some frozen peach pies use shelf-stable vegetable shortening for better freshness, adding (partially) hydrogenated fats (aka trans fats) that are harmful to your heart.

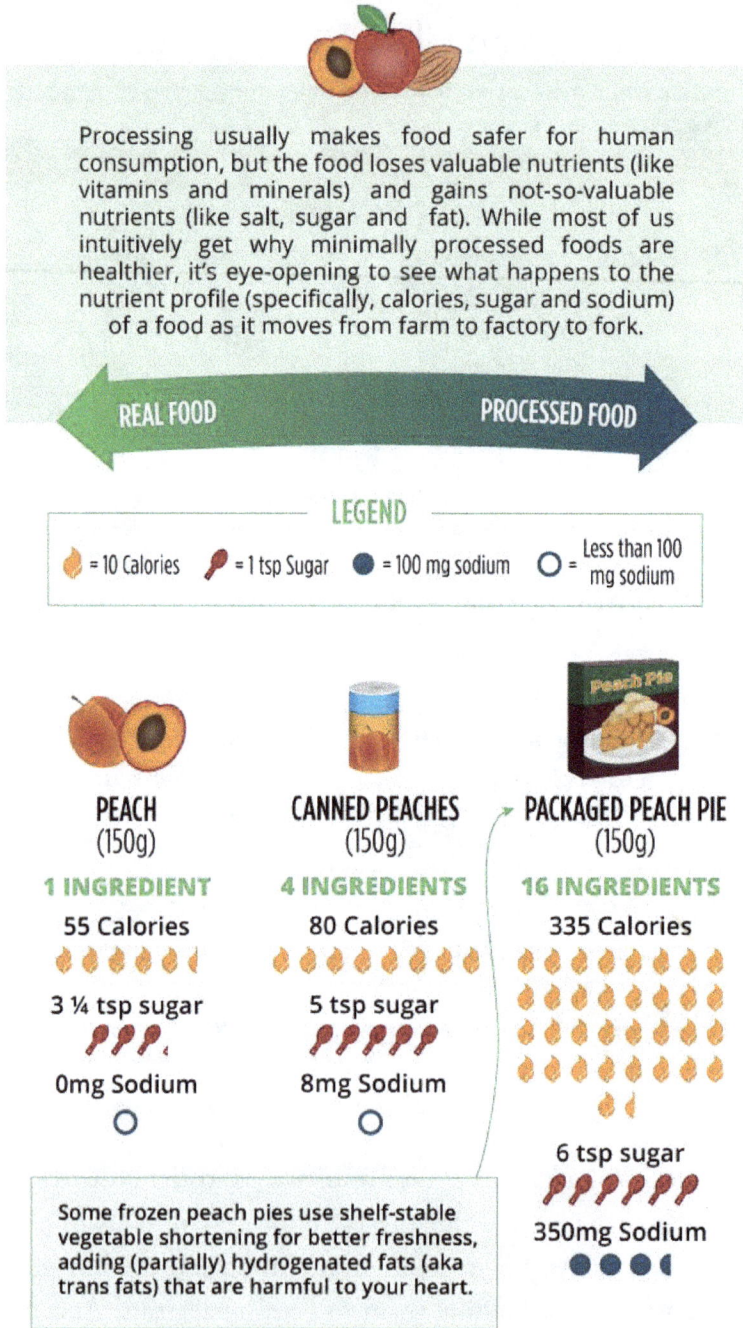

Diagram 3: An Intuitive Guide to What Ultra-Processing Does to Real Food [24]

---

[24] Diagram source: https://mindovermunch.com/blog/are-processed-foods-bad/, (site visited on 9/3/19). Note this website has a much longer and very useful infographic from which this image was drawn. For those who like to assimilate their information visually, I strongly recommend looking at the images at the end of the article.

When you eat out, try to limit yourself to restaurants that slow-cook healthy food. Yes, this means avoiding fast food like the plague. When you shop to cook for yourself (remember Rule 4: cook for yourself), buy things that look like they would at the farmer's market or the butcher's shop or dairy. If it comes in a box or colorful package or freezer bag, if it's in the center aisle at the grocery store, placed at your kids' eye level so that they will jump up and down to get you to buy it, alarms should sound, and you should go straight to the ingredient list (or as far away as possible!). Please note that one of the tricks that the food industry plays on us, with the help of the FDA, is to put misleading labels on food, like "Natural" or "Low Cholesterol" or "Fat Free."[25]

Ultra-processed food is made from 3 highly processed ingredients

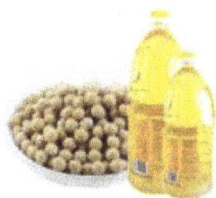
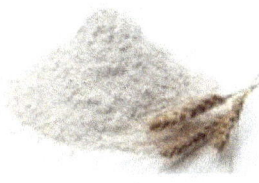
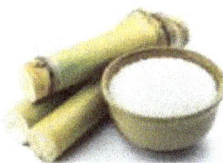

Chemically extracted seed oils, soy oil most common

Refined (bran and germ removed, bleached) cereal grains ground very fine

Sugar is extracted from sugar cane, refined, cleaned and dried

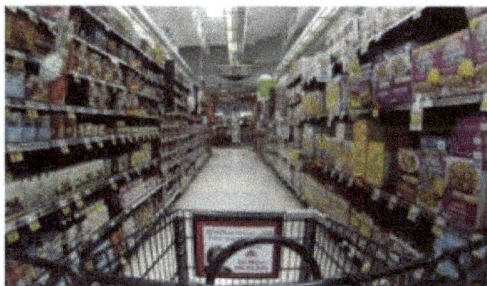
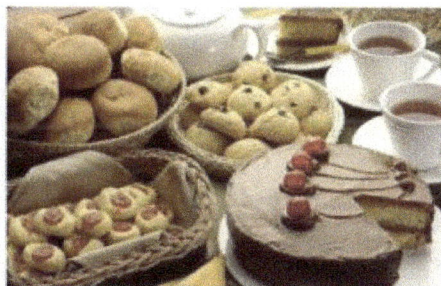

We buy some

We make some

Diagram 4: What Makes "Food" Products Ultra-Processed is What's In Them, Not Where They Were Made or Bought.[26]

---

[25] One useful source for deciphering misleading labels is the FoodPrint website and app. They are primarily focused on issues of environmental sustainability as they relate to food (the idea is to calculate the FoodPrint of your diet in the same way that you calculate the footprint of your other consumption and lifestyle habits), but also have a wealth of information about eating healthy and ethical food, including a Food Label Guide. (see < https://foodprint.org/eating-sustainably/food-label-guide/ >).

[26] Diagram source: http://juliannetaylornutrition.com/2018/04/the-cookie-how-exactly-does-it-contribute-to-overeating-and-obesity/ (site visited 9/3/19).

Reading the label is no substitute for reading the ingredient list. If the product contains ingredients you or your grandmother has never heard of, stay away. Such food products are not so much grown as engineered. They are engineered to be highly addictive and to displace your healthy appetite for unprocessed food with intense cravings for ultra-processed food (this is what I feel when I drive past a donut shop or ice cream store). Once you are hooked on highly processed food, you are on a path that leads quickly to weight gain, obesity, and not long after that, diabetes, heart disease, and other awful health disorders.

If you're already hooked, it's going to take a lot of willpower, understanding, patience, and help from your friends and family to change your diet, because our entire food system is designed to keep you addicted. But it is possible—I have done it myself, and counseled thousands of patients at my clinics on how to change their diet, with a very high success rate and results that last for years. (More on this in the diet section.)

The first and most important trick is to learn to look at food differently. Don't simply ask, "Do I want that?" or "Wouldn't it be yummy?" Instead, consider: Is it real food? Is it going to sustain me with the nutrients I need to grow, stay strong, and survive? Or is it a "food" product that has been engineered by an industry that makes its profits by getting me addicted to something they know is not just bad for me but leads to obesity and disease? Is it more important that it tastes good or that it poisons me and rewires the reward circuitry of my brain so that I want it instead of real food?

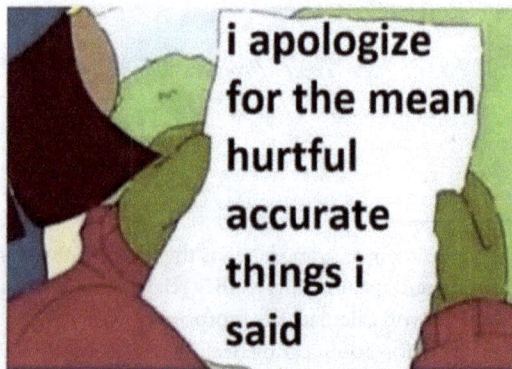

I know—not the most fun series of questions to ask yourself, but this form of critical thinking is vital if you want to live a long, healthy, productive, and fulfilling life. If you think about the questions in the right way, the answers are easy, even if resisting the allure of junk food won't be at first. But as you start to clean up your diet, the cravings will become less intense, and you will start to desire and enjoy real food more. Eventually, your body and brain will associate real food with health and well-being, and ultra-processed food with the immediate discomfort and lethargy it often causes. Once that's happened, you will have rewired your food reward system so that you really want what is good for you.

Rule 2: Eat Organic Food

The "organic" label is one of the few somewhat meaningful labels in the food industry today, and numerous studies show that organic foods are nutrient rich and generally do not contain much of the toxicity associated with industrial agriculture. It is not a perfect system, and there are efforts underway to improve it (be on the lookout for the emerging "regenerative-organic" label), but many nutritionists and environmentalists regard it as a bare minimum—a floor below which you shouldn't sink. To understand why, consider how toxic the nonorganic food system is. A majority of what the industrial agricultural system produces cannot be consumed without being ultra-processed using industrial chemistry or supplemented with unhealthy additives (e.g., sugar, preservatives). Such foods are grown with petroleum-based fertilizers so powerful that they quickly destroy the natural biome of the soil, depleting crops grown this way of the nutrient density they take up from healthy soil.

Ultra-processed food vs unprocessed food

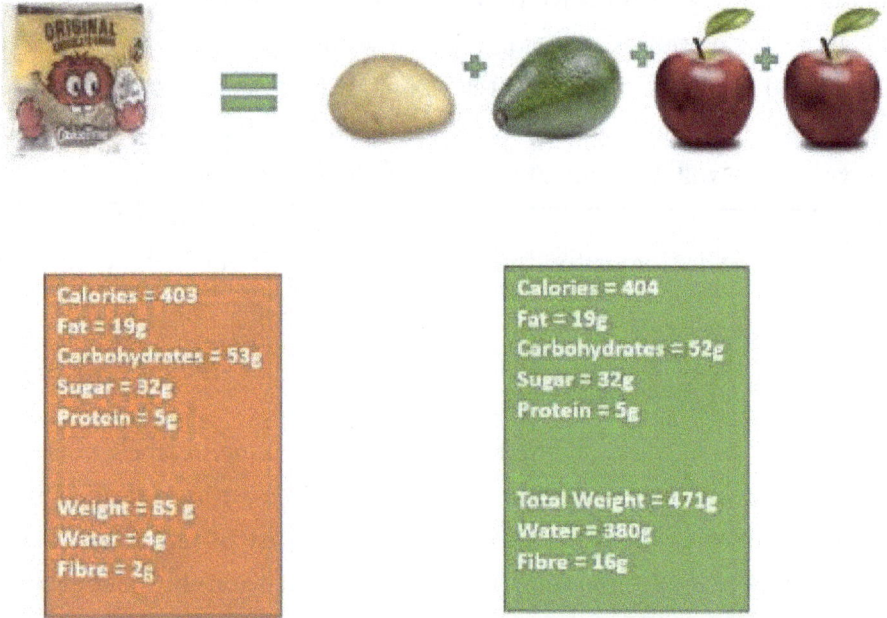

Calories = 403	Calories = 404
Fat = 19g	Fat = 19g
Carbohydrates = 53g	Carbohydrates = 52g
Sugar = 32g	Sugar = 32g
Protein = 5g	Protein = 5g
Weight = 85 g	Total Weight = 471g
Water = 4g	Water = 380g
Fibre = 2g	Fibre = 16g

Diagram 5: Ultra-processed Foods and Calories—Which Do You Think is More Filling?[27]

The result: You will be better satiated (full) when eating less of a meal made from organic produce, meats, and dairy than when eating larger portions of the same meal made with nonorganic food, because there will be more nutrients per ounce in the organic meal. In short, organic food belonging to NOVA Group 1 is the best kind of real food. According to a recent meta-analysis of many other studies, organic dairy and meat contain about 50% more omega-3 fatty acids. The study authors note: "Omega-3s are linked to reductions in cardiovascular disease, improved neurological development and function, and better immune function."[28]

Another study found that organic crops have substantially higher concentrations of a range of antioxidants and other potentially beneficial compounds—for instance, 50% more anthocyanins and flavonols than conventional crops. These compounds have

---

[27] http://juliannetaylornutrition.com/2018/04/the-cookie-how-exactly-does-it-contribute-to-overeating-and-obesity/ (site visited 9/3/19)

[28] Średnicka-Tober, Dominika et al. "Higher PUFA and n-3 PUFA, conjugated linoleic acid, α-tocopherol and iron, but lower iodine and selenium concentrations in organic milk: a systematic literature review and meta- and redundancy analyses." *The British Journal of Nutrition* vol. 115,6 (2016): 1043-60. doi:10.1017/S0007114516000349.

anti-inflammatory effects that protect cells from damage, which can help fend off disease.[29] Yet another study concludes that organic foods are higher in phenolic phytonutrients, which are thought to be the source of the benefits ascribed to eating fruits and vegetables. Organic fruits and vegetables had between 19% and 69% more of a variety of these antioxidant compounds than nonorganic produce.[30] In summary, organic foods are simply healthier and do what we want real food to do: sustain, nourish, and protect us, allowing our bodies to function well so that we can grow and thrive.

Nonorganic foods, on the other hand, often contain toxins from the pesticides used to grow them and have a higher incidence of causing foodborne diseases. They also contribute to antibiotic-resistant superbugs.[31] One of my favorite stories comes from Michael Pollan's *Omnivore's Dilemma*, in which he recounts visiting a farm growing potatoes for McDonald's french fries. The pesticide used was so toxic that the farmer huddled in a concrete bunker while it was applied and could not send humans into the field for days after the pesticide had been applied without risking poisoning them. Sounds more like chemical warfare than agriculture, right? Well, the modern pesticides, it turns out, arose from the need to repurpose chemical weapons technology at the end of World War II. The pesticide used at the potato farm in question, like many others, was "systemic," meaning it didn't just stay on the skin or surface level of the potato but permeated the entire vegetable and stayed in it at poisonous levels until after it had been harvested and off-gassed for months! Appetizing, no?

Moral of the story: avoid conventional or nonorganic produce, meat, and dairy if you can.

Rule 3: Eat Meat and Dairy Sparingly, if you eat it at all, and eat meat and dairy from pasture-raised animals

The meat-rich diet that many in the developed world eat is quite new, and frankly our digestive tracts and body chemistry are ill-suited to process that much meat. This reality is one of the reasons for the rapid increase in obesity, heart disease, diabetes, and other

---

[29] Barański, Marcin et al. "Higher antioxidant and lower cadmium concentrations and lower incidence of pesticide residues in organically grown crops: a systematic literature review and meta-analyses." *The British Journal of Nutrition* vol. 112,5 (2014): 794-811. doi:10.1017/S0007114514001366.

[30] Greger, M. FACLM, "Organic versus Conventional: Which has More Nutrients?", NutritionFacts.Org, April 13th, 2017, (https://nutritionfacts.org/2017/04/13/organic-versus-conventional-which-has-more-nutrients/) (site visited on 9/1/2019).

[31] For a balanced overview, see: Mie, Axel et al. "Human health implications of organic food and organic agriculture: a comprehensive review." *Environmental health: a global access science source* vol. 16,1 111. 27 Oct. 2017, doi:10.1186/s12940-017-0315-4

diseases plaguing populations all over the world, especially those lacking strong indigenous food cultures. If you eat meat, adopt an approach that monitors and limits the amount you eat, such as Mark Bittman's Vegan Before 6:00 (VB6) diet or the Johns Hopkins' Center for a Livable Future's Meatless Monday program.[32] Meat and dairy from animals that are not pasture raised is unhealthy for us. Cows are ruminants, which means they have special stomachs that allow them to ferment grass that most other animals cannot eat. But when you confine an animal built to eat grass to a feedlot and give it a grain-based diet instead (remember, we overproduce corn and soy), it gets sick and has to be pumped full of antibiotics and other medicines. This kind of farming is awful for the environment and a major source of methane, a powerful greenhouse gas (by some estimates, roughly 20% of all greenhouse gases can be traced back to the industrial food system), but it is also bad for us. Residuals of antibiotics and other medicines remain in the products of lot-fed animals. There is a significantly higher incidence of foodborne illness from these products, and food made with these ingredients is less nutritious. Do yourself a favor and look for grass-fed, free-range, and organic meat and dairy.

Rule 4: Cook Your Own Food (and cook slow food)

Like everything else on this list, this is not a moral absolute but a good rule of thumb for healthy eating. It is also one of the hardest rules to integrate into your life if you are used to eating out a lot. However, it is a solid foundation for the first three rules, because it's very hard to eat real food—organic and responsibly grown produce, meat, and dairy—and to reduce meat consumption if you don't shop for and cook your own food. This is especially the case if you eat at the ultra-processed, highly addictive, nutrient-weak, saturated fat–heavy fare you get at fast food restaurants. That's why I strongly recommend making the time and acquiring the knowledge necessary to cook the majority of your food.

Helpful resources abound in the books at the beginning of this section, and the cookbooks written by Mark Bittman, or any of the Moosewood cookbooks, can be a good place to start. Other good places to turn are the Slow Food movement, founded in Italy over 30 years ago by Carlo Petrini (see slowfood.com), and Alice Waters' Edible Schoolyard programs (including the wonderful annual lecture series at UC Berkeley, Edible Education 101). There are many other programs, so be sure to see what's available near you. (I am lucky to have the Stone Barns Center for Food and Agriculture in my own backyard.)

---

[32] See Bittman, *VB6: Eat Vegan Before 6:00 to Lose Weight and Restore Your Health…for Good*, (New York: Clarkson Potter, 2013); and <https://www.meatlessmonday.com/>.

HEDONIC EATING AND ULTRA-PROCESSED FOODS—A *DEAD*-END PATH TO HAPPINESS

To internalize the above four lessons, you don't need a full understanding of body and brain chemistry, but I know some readers will be curious to know why these four rules work. Robert Lustig has a thorough discussion of these issues in his books *Fat Chance* and *The Hacking of the American Mind*, but here I'll provide just an introduction to illustrate how these rules can transform your relationship with food, making it much easier not only to lose weight and then maintain your weight loss but also to thrive physically and mentally in a long, productive life.

One of the themes that Lustig emphasizes is that our entire food industry preys on us by trying to get us to engage in hedonic eating—that is, eating for rewards beyond those intrinsic to eating healthy, delicious food. Hedonic hunger (or hyperphagia) is "the drive to eat to obtain pleasure in the absence of an energy deficit" or physical need for caloric intake.[33] Hedonic eating habits can arise, in part, from being exposed to advertising campaigns that associate specific food and drink brands with status, coolness, health, and happiness. The irony is that almost all of the brands that employ these marketing strategies produce products that are, in fact, unhealthy and can, over the long term, increase the risk of diseases that will certainly diminish your happiness.

Individuals who eat only for the pleasure boost may be compensating for other things that are lacking in their life. (In chapter 7, I will address the need to have sources of genuine happiness and contentment in order to be healthy during a long life.) Physical health and its relation to eating well is also connected to the themes of mental and psychological health emphasized in the first chapter's discussion about the need to have a realistic and healthy self-image.

A trillion-dollar industry is spending tens of billions of dollars a year to convince you to eat unhealthy food for the wrong reasons. Much of this advertising is aimed at children (think sugary cereal and soda ads) who do not yet have the cognitive capacities required to understand what those commercials are trying to do to them. The ultra-processed junk and fast foods in question do give you a dopamine rush, because they're loaded with sugar, fats, and salts that lead the body to release this powerful neurotransmitter. This leads

---

[33] In addition to Lustig's books, cited above, see: Nicole M. Avena, *Hedonic Eating: How the Pleasure of Food Affects Our Brains and Behavior*, (Oxford: Oxford University Press, 2015).

researchers to suggest that food addiction is comparable to drug and gambling addiction, since the same neural pathways and behavior patterns are at work in each of these cases.[34]

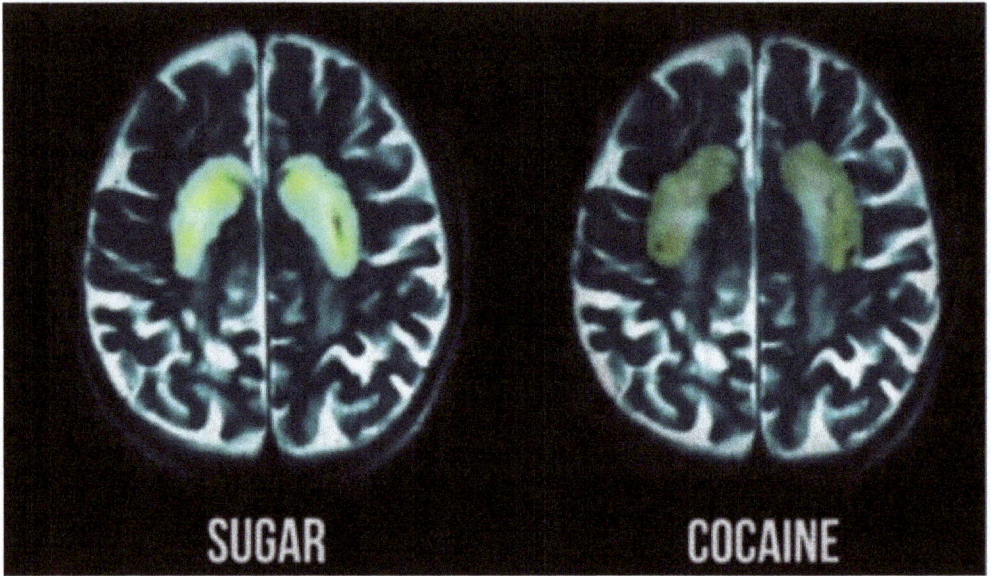

Diagram 6: This is Your Brain on Sugar (Note that the dopamine surge from sugar is even more intense than that from the other white powder.)[35]

The food systems of most developed countries make bad food abundantly available and more affordable. This is abundantly clear if you measure in terms of calories per dollar. (The cheapest source of calories at almost every grocery store in America is soda.) Note that the opposite is true if you measure in terms of public health expenditures to treat ailments and diseases that can be traced directly to our bad diets. As a society and individuals, we ultimately pay for the costs of our unhealthy diet when we foot the bill to treat the ill health and disease it produces.

The agricultural industrial complex spends tens of billions of dollars a year trying to get all of us hooked on bad food. We consume bad food because it's cheap, easy, and sold to us as cool, healthy, fun, and the source of happiness. It rewires our food reward circuitry, the neurochemistry of the limbic system of the brain, making us crave more and more bad food. Once you appreciate this, you may conclude, as I have, that the food industry is a lot like the tobacco and alcohol industries. Both their products and their advertising should be carefully regulated for the sake of public health. Fast food, junk food, and soda

---

[34] See Lowe, M. R. and Butryn, M. L., "Hedonic hunger: A new dimension of appetite?", *Physiology & Behavior*, Vol. 91, July 24, 2007, pp. 432-39.
[35] https://mindovermunch.com/blog/are-processed-foods-bad/, (site visited on 9/3/19).

commercials directed at children should be illegal, and those addressed at adults should come with clear warnings about how unhealthy the food actually is and the long-term health risks of regular consumption. Further, these industries should be taxed so that they have to bear the true public health cost of the diseases caused by the diet they market, just as cigarettes are now taxed to pay for the treatment of lung cancer and to discourage consumption.

A recent study led by Kevin Hall took a group of subjects, divided them into two groups that ate essentially the same diet, with one important exception. The first group was fed a diet composed entirely of unprocessed food, and the second got a diet of exclusively ultra-processed food products. After a couple weeks, the researchers switched the two groups, so the first switched from eating unprocessed food to eating ultra-processed food, and the second switched from eating ultra-processed food to eating unprocessed food. In both instances, those who ate real food ate fewer calories and lost weight, while those who ate ultra-processed food products ate more calories and gained weight. (See the diagram below reproduced from Hall's study.)

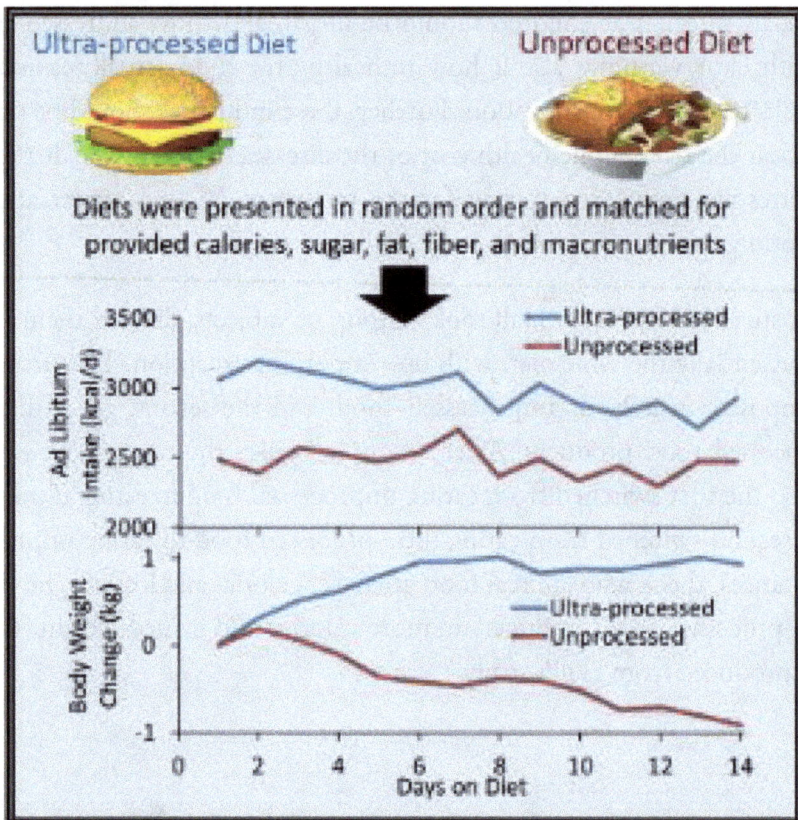

Diagram 7: The Effects on Weight of Eating Real Food vs. Ultra-Processed Products[36]

What in the world is going on here? Feed people as much unprocessed food as they want to eat for two weeks, and they eat less and lose weight? Then feed the same people the same diet but of ultra-processed foods, and they eat more and gain weight? This is clear evidence of the central lesson of this chapter. Bad food isn't just bad for you—it changes the wiring of the food reward system in your brain so that you crave and eat more of it. In this case, Hall notes that the production of the body's natural appetite-suppressing hormone, PYY, increased during the unprocessed diet, and production of the hunger hormone, ghrelin, decreased, unlike in the ultra-processed diet. This explains why you eat ultra-processed foods more quickly than unprocessed foods—they don't contain the nutrients and compounds that tell your brain that your body is getting what it needs, so you remain hungrier for longer and eat more.

---

[36] From Kevin D. Hall,, et. al., "Ultra-Processed Diets Cause Excess Calorie Intake and Weight Gain: An Inpatient Randomized Controlled Trial of Ad Libitum Food Intake," *Cell Metabolism* 30, 67–77 July 2, 2019.

What is the takeaway from all of this? You should view fast, junk, and ultra-processed food the same way you would view a highly addictive drug. Regulate your consumption accordingly. You need to want the right food (real food)—and want it for the right reason: because it tastes good when it is well prepared, satisfies your hunger without leading to further cravings, and sustains you with nutrients that lead your body to function and thrive. When you think about what food to eat, ask yourself: Is it good for me? Will it nourish and support my body to live with health and vitality? A question of secondary importance is: Will it give me pleasure? Sure, we get some pleasure from eating, but this cannot be our primary motivation for eating what we eat—that's hedonic eating. If you look to food primarily for pleasure, it almost certainly means that there are other pieces missing from your life.

Finally, if you want to eat *this particular brand* of food product (especially when it's brightly packaged, marketed in a sophisticated multimedia campaign, and found at eye level in the center of your grocery store) because you think it's cool or confers a certain status or will make you attractive to some person or group you want to impress, you are being suckered by the food industry. With a bit of deliberate, careful thought, you can recognize this as a fool's errand. There is good news in all of this: These lessons are not that hard to learn, the rules aren't hard to apply, and once you establish good food habits, you will no longer crave bad food nearly as much. You will see the commercials for what they are: efforts like those of the tobacco industry to get you hooked on substances that alter your brain and body chemistry and lead to ill health and disease.

LESSON LEARNED? X-RAY YOUR PLATE

With this brief explanation on the effects of ultra-processed food, I hope you have a better understanding of why following the four, relatively simple rules of thumb above are an essential foundation to lifelong health and flourishing. Occasional lapses will happen, and that's fine. (You don't have to completely forswear ice cream or turn down the occasional meal out with friends or family!) If you follow these guidelines most of the time, you are well on your way to a healthier diet and long-term well-being and vitality.

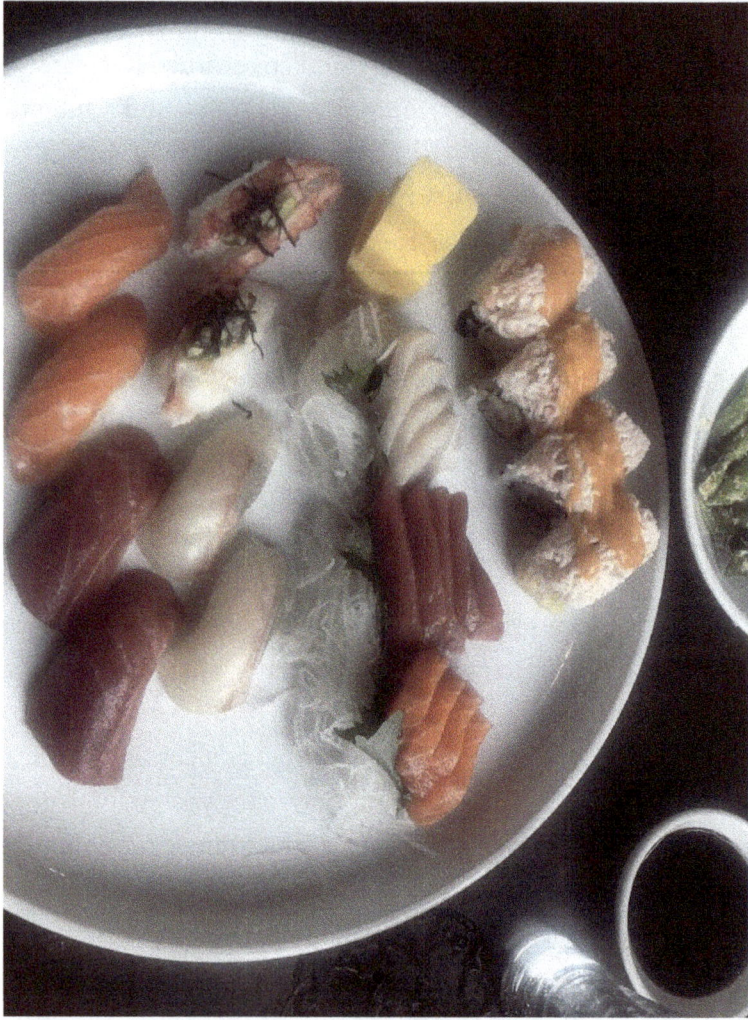

Let me shamelessly toot my own horn here for a moment by stating that my medical practice has one of the highest rates of successful weight reduction results, with clients maintaining weight loss for over two years. I know diets inside out (because I've tried them!), and I have learned to guide my clients and help them know how to eat. I fought on-and-off weight gain for years because of chronic stress. I was a single mother, working as a doctor running two private medical businesses. I was a classic yo-yo dieter. But I am so grateful for this experience because it taught me how to eat well and learn what works for my body. Experience can be a harsh but reliable teacher.

So how can you apply these rules to your life? One simple practice is to "x-ray" your plate before you dig in to eat a meal. Ask the following questions of the food sitting in front of you:

1. Do you know where everything on your plate comes from?
2. Do you know why it's there?
   - What does it do for or to you?
   - Does it contribute to your health?
   - Does it have any side effects?
3. Do you know how it was prepared and what went into it (e.g., the type of oil, how much sugar)?
4. Are you concerned about anything else related to your food?
   - What is the environmental impact and sustainability of what you're eating?
   - What are the ethical implications of the way in which the food was produced? Were there other people involved in making the food, and were they treated decently?
   - What is the impact on animal health and welfare of the food you're eating?

If you can answer these questions, you have x-rayed your plate and know much more about what you're about to put in your mouth and what it's likely to do to your body.

X-raying your plate and applying the above four rules really doesn't amount to a diet. I haven't suggested that you limit the number of calories you consume or emphasized having a diet that is low or high in certain kinds of foods beyond eating real food and avoiding ultra-processed food products. Some thoughts on more specific diets and medical weight reduction procedures are covered in another chapter. If you've already fallen victim to the industrial food system and are overweight, obese, or suffering other negative effects from eating, then you may need those diet approaches.

But before getting to that, it is essential to emphasize that healthy eating is the foundation of human health and long-term physical and mental vitality, and the guidelines for healthy eating are really quite simple—as simple as the four rules above. Remember Kevin Hall's study? Give people as much unprocessed real food as they want, and they will eat less and lose weight. Give the same people ultra-processed food, and they will eat more and gain weight. These results show the rules above should form the cornerstone of any diet you may want to try.

The rules are not hard, though following them often is. Don't be hard on yourself or think it's all a simple matter of willpower. A huge industry is trying to get you to violate the rules, and the government is backing them up. You will need patience, support, and understanding to change the way you eat. But the reward is immense: You will be healthier, more attractive, more energetic, less tempted, and eventually even disgusted by bad food.

EXERCISE—NOTE TO SELF

There is no chapter in this book on exercise, but that is not meant to diminish its significance. Rather, it reflects the limits of my expertise as a doctor. But I will conclude this chapter with a brief postscript on exercise.

Just as you cannot exercise your way out of a bad diet, you cannot eat your way to good health without also exercising. I am not the one to tell you which exercise program to adopt, and fortunately, there's no shortage of good books and experts to help you where I can't. I will tell you that you should be active every day, preferably every hour.

Walking, even if it's just for five minutes at a time, restores circulation and boosts your metabolism and organ functioning. It's also good for your mind, as it restores clarity of thought. You should do a form of exercise that involves greater exertion several (at least four) times a week. The aim should be to elevate your heart rate, as well as to strengthen your muscles and sharpen your balance and reflexes. I am a fan of high intensity interval training (HIIT) and in wearing a fitness device that monitors your activity and nudges you when you are inactive for too long.

If you set concrete goals, note your successes, and monitor the effects of exercise on your body, mind, and energy level for even just a few weeks, I believe you will quickly notice that you are stronger, more energetic, and more productive. And let's remember that the point is to have a Mercedes engine inside your Mercedes body. If you exercise regularly, you will age better and be less prone to diseases, falls, and physical deterioration. Seeing so many suffering geriatric patients who hadn't properly cared for themselves earlier in life is what led me into anti-aging medicine in the first place.

CHAPTER 6

WEIGHT LOSS WITHOUT FAT SHAMING

If you have flipped to this chapter on weight loss without first reading the preceding chapter on food, my plea to you is to stop right now and go back to chapter 5—especially the crash course on food education. Seriously, take it from someone who learned this lesson the hard way and has more than a decade's worth of experience in managing patients' weight loss and obesity management programs. For the sake of your health and longevity, not to mention your overall well-being, productivity, and flourishing, I want to help you not only to lose weight but also to keep it off, and to do that, you may benefit from some of the procedures, medications, and diets I describe in this chapter. But you will not sustain permanent weight loss with its real physical and psychological health benefits unless you also educate yourself about food and adopt a healthy, lifelong approach to eating. So go read chapter 5 if you haven't already. I can wait.

Since you've now read the previous chapter, you know I don't blame you if you're overweight or obese. I blame the food industrial complex and the mainstream media and government in the U.S. for the obesity epidemic. The food supply in this country and many other countries is full of ultra-processed, highly addictive foods that are borderline toxic, and literally billions of dollars a year are spent to keep you addicted to this crap. And within my own profession, as we will see below, most health insurance policies do not cover the most effective weight loss and obesity treatments.

If you are overweight or obese, you are largely the victim of a public health and public policy failure, and of a culture that does too little to call attention to and address the attendant crises. Don't get me wrong—you personally will suffer adverse health consequences that may shorten your life and decrease your productivity and contentment while you're alive. That's bad enough. I see no reason to blame you further when the deck is so badly stacked against you. Instead, I want to help you and share the most important lessons for getting you on a better path.

But some of us, myself included, aren't lucky enough to just start eating better, exercising more, and watching our bodies heal themselves and return to a healthy weight. That doesn't mean that the rules from chapter 5 aren't the foundation for healthy eating and ultimately lifelong health and well-being. They are. But you may need to do more at first, especially if you've been feeding your body junk for too long. The advice contained in this chapter is for you.

LIFE IN THE TIME OF COOLSCULPTING AND WEIGHT LOSS PILLS

I often get asked what diet pill is best for losing weight. There are a bunch of FDA-approved weight loss pills on the market that have brand names such as Qsymia, Contrave, Belviq, and phentermine but are not covered by health insurance, so people usually have to buy them out of pocket. This is more than an inconvenience because, for reasons explained in the previous chapter, excess weight and obesity are at the center of an epidemic, and most people really can't afford to purchase these expensive medications. Furthermore, the medications require monitoring and blood work, which adds to the expense. In the absence of better health care and support systems, people are stacking on the pound and suffering the consequences of obesity and related illnesses, diseases, and comorbidities.

This lack of healthcare intervention and governmental support leads many people to use over-the-counter (OTC) fad products that are not even regulated by the FDA. In my practice, I meet people with side effects from OTC products that frequently cause problems as diverse as heart palpitations, hair loss, and increased urination. Should you try OTC products? My answer is always, "Please don't." They may cause harm if taken without your doctor's knowledge and supervision.

Most diets are not covered by your health insurance, and I know it's tempting to try the products you find at the drugstore or online to get that skinnier version of you—especially since you are paying out of pocket. But slow down, think carefully, and don't be fooled again! It's not only much safer but also much more effective to speak to a doctor well versed in obesity management (often your primary care doctor) or a nutritionist who works in tandem with a doctor.

I am a firm believer that your primary care doctor must treat your excess weight or obesity as symptoms of progressive disease. But there is a shortage of primary care doctors in the U.S., and many of them are so overworked and discouraged that they don't take the time for this essential healthcare intervention. You should demand that your primary care doctor assist you with weight management and dietary health or refer you to someone who will. If he or she won't, get a new doctor! Roughly 53,000 more primary care doctors will be needed in the U.S. by the year 2025 just to fulfill routine needs of a growing and aging population.[37] And the patient load on primary care doctors has increased significantly over the last decade because of a decrease in reimbursements from health insurance. These added stressors have caused worse patient care and physician burnout.

These conditions among trained healthcare providers have given an unfair advantage to less skilled and voodoo providers like naturopaths who have limited training and don't go through pre-med programs, testing, medical school, or residency training programs in accredited hospitals or medical clinics before managing people's health. The fact that FDA-regulated products are also not covered by insurance puts the medications that have solid scientific data and safety profiles in direct competition with the cheaper naturopathic, unverified voodoo bullshit (also not covered by insurance, but often of comparable cost or less expensive).

This leads me to an important problem faced by science and healthcare today: the return of witchcraft and voodoo medicine in the form of inflated claims related to naturopathy and homeopathy. I strongly believe that you put your health at risk if you turn to unregulated OTC products for weight loss (or any other health-related issue) or put your faith in practitioners who rely on them.

In Arizona, the naturopathic board was able to get state licensors to agree to let them call themselves doctors and even prescribe controlled medications. To me, this looks just like a developing country's healthcare system, where anyone can go anywhere to buy anything without state regulation. People are left to fend for themselves. Since the average time a naturopath spends is over 1.5 hours with a patient in one sitting, they are able to make strong personal connections, something far too often lacking in traditional medicine. But many naturo- and homeopaths' training and health management skills remain weak, and too often the treatments they recommend prove questionable at best.[38]

To be perfectly clear, I am a big fan of botanicals and believe there is much to be learned from non-Western and indigenous medicine. So, I'm not opposed to naturopathy as such. In fact, I study and recommend approaches and remedies that come out of these traditions

---

[37] Petterson, S. M. 1, Liaw, W. R., Phillips, R. L. Jr, Rabin D. L., Meyers, D. S., and Bazemore, A. W., "Projecting US primary care physician workforce needs: 2010-2025," Ann Fam Med. 2012 Nov-Dec; 10(6):503-9. doi: 10.1370/afm.1431

[38] Please refer to Britt Hermes blog at http://naturopathicdiaries.com for a first hand account that may give you some second thoughts and perhaps even goosebumps about naturopathic medicine. For a book length study, see *Simon Singh and Edzard Ernst, Trick or Treatment?: The Undeniable Facts about Alternative Medicine*, (New York: W. W. Norton, 2009).

and wish more doctors and medical schools were better versed in them. What concerns me, and what I am warning you against, is relying on homeo- and naturopaths instead of doctors when it comes to medical treatment of a broad range of health concerns, from weight loss to disease treatment. A truly responsible homeo- or naturopath will advise to always also consult with a well-trained medical doctor. That is my advice, too.

The FDA-approved medications that are routinely given to pacify the appetite centers in your brain are usually fraught with potential side effects. Medications like phentermine, Qsymia, Contrave, and Belviq have shown a 5–10% short-term decrease in weight, but most people gain back the lost weight once they go off the meds, unless they change their lifestyles at the same time. In my medical practice, I have found it considerably more effective to avoid these meds or at least combine them with treatments such as CoolSculpting to hasten results. I combine medical treatment with sound dietary advice and informal counseling designed to help my patients develop positive body image goals, sound diets, and exercise regimens. The combined result is high rates of successful weight loss maintained for at least two years. But while this combined approach to weight loss shows real promise, few of these services are covered by most health insurance plans. Some "limousine" plans will pay for a portion of the medication, but in most cases, my clients usually pay for them out of their own pockets.

BARIATRIC SURGERY DOS AND DON'TS

Some health insurance *will* cover bariatric surgery, a surgical approach to food addiction and obesity that involves reducing the area of food absorption by removing portions of your gut.

I simply don't recommend bariatric surgery procedures unless a client's body mass index (BMI), a medical measure of patient's weight relative to their height, has become so high that the client cannot manage weight with diet, nonsurgical techniques, or other approaches that are contraindicated.

There is an increasingly better understanding of the gut's role in generating and regulating emotions, but emotional side effects in people who undergo bariatric surgery are common. Ideally, candidates will go through a psychological assessment before undergoing this procedure and demonstrate that they are not addicts. But barring people with a serious metabolic disorder, almost no one gains enough weight to be a candidate for bariatric surgery without being a food addict. Many of my clients who chose to get bariatric surgery for better health have developed emotional and psychological problems since their surgeries. In the absence of good psychiatric support covered by their health insurance, they usually go untreated or suffer poor treatment.

Although I consider this procedure a last resort, other doctors may recommend surgery for people with a BMI of 35. (I prefer 45.) For people in the lower BMI range, there is still hope that nonsurgical methods will work. Until neuroscience advances to the point where we can treat hunger neurochemically (and without severe mental health–related side effects), it will be simply too difficult for some people to lose weight and keep it off. But please consider the various procedures and diets listed below before turning to bariatric surgery.

mcdonalds ✔   •••

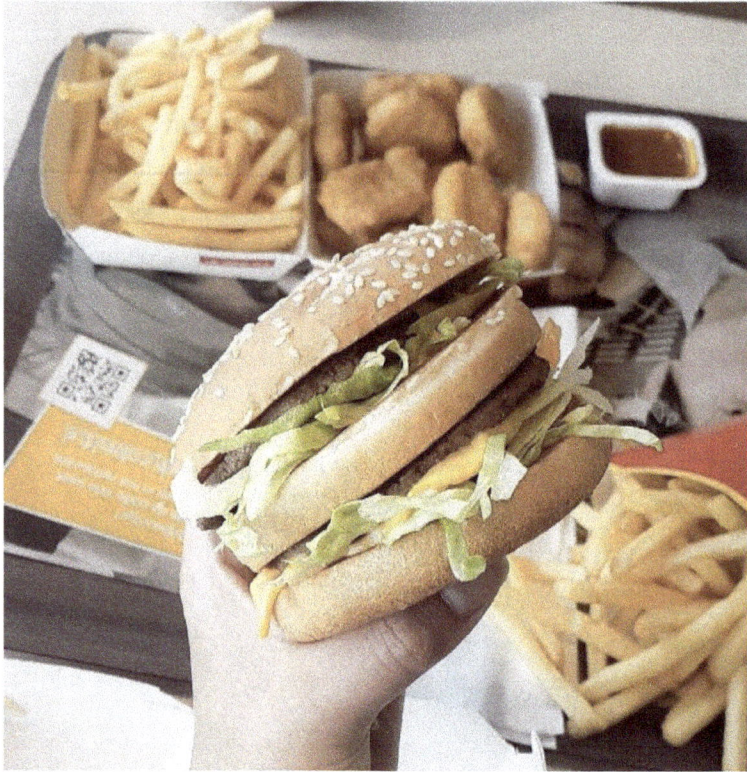

♡   ⬭   ◁   ⬚

38,090 likes

mcdonalds Some people only measure life in two time periods: before their first #BigMac and everything else that comes after.

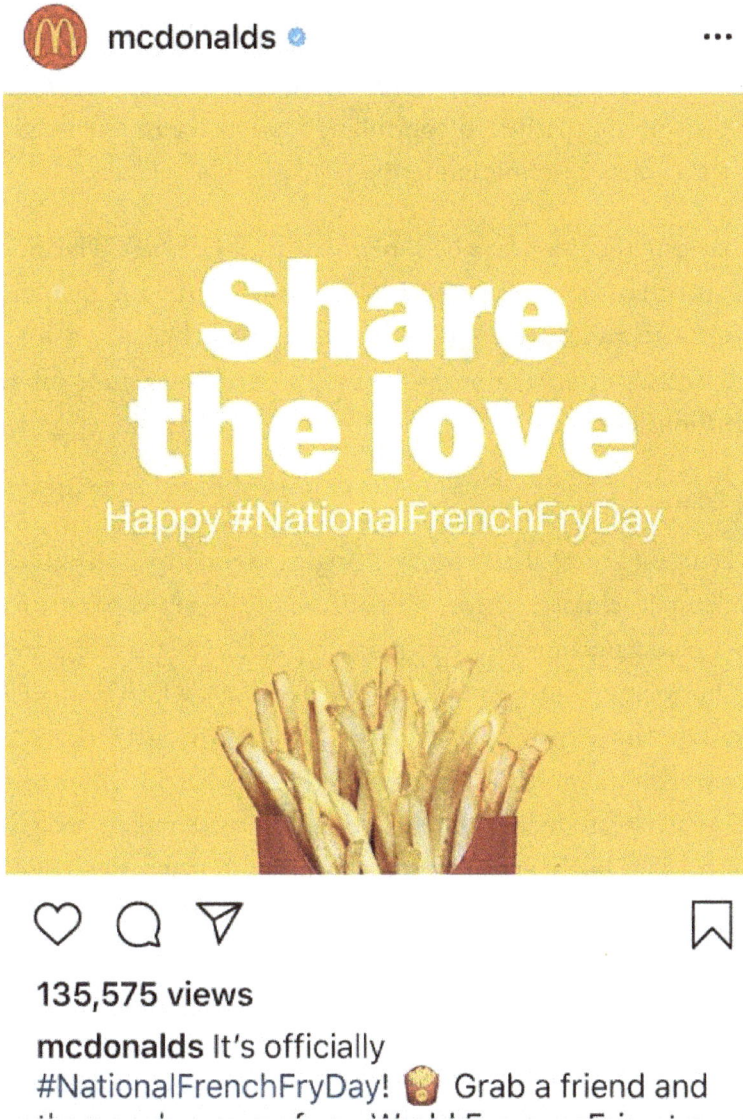

mcdonalds ✓   •••

Share the love
Happy #NationalFrenchFryDay

♡ ◯ ▽   ⊓

135,575 views

mcdonalds It's officially
#NationalFrenchFryDay! 🍟 Grab a friend and

OBESITY AND WEIGHT LOSS MANAGEMENT

The first step in obesity management should be to lose the weight of other people's opinions.

The remainder of this chapter will focus on nonsurgical, primarily dietary approaches to weight loss, or "weight release," as I recently heard someone call it. (Language matters, and how we phrase our problems is important.) This is not a diet book, and I am not a dietician, so my approach will not be systematic. Instead, I'll offer a brief tour of some of the approaches I am most familiar with and have been most effective. I'm also not an advocate for a particular diet or approach, though I will evaluate what I view as the strengths and weaknesses of the ones I describe. Specifically, I will discuss four main families of diets or approaches to controlling food intake to lose weight: ketogenic diets, calorie restriction diets, intermittent fasting, and plant-based diets.

Before we navigate the trees, let's be sure not to lose the forest. The most important thing is to find a diet that allows you to get to a healthy weight and then maintain it—not by going on and off various diets (I, too, was a proverbial yo-yo for a while), but by permanently altering your relationship to food so that you get the calories you need from healthy, nutritious sources.

Ketogenic Diets

What is a ketogenic diet? This diet was originally used to treat intractable (difficult to control) epilepsy in children before anti-seizure meds gained popularity. Keto dieters eat foods with a moderate amount of protein, few carbs (20g to 50g), and lots of fats. This makes your body enter a ketogenic state (called ketosis), which is when it shifts to burning energy from fats rather than carbohydrates. Most Americans eat carbohydrate-rich diets, which affects brain chemistry since glucose is burned as fuel. But in high-fat ketogenic diets, the liver starts producing ketone bodies, and these replace the glucose in the brain. There is a myth that the brain only runs on glucose, but actually it also runs very well on beta-hydroxybutyrate (part of a ketone body structure). Ketone bodies are basically a chemical that our liver produces when it burns fat. Each gram of fat is equal to nine calories.

9 Fruits to Eat
On Keto Diet
@help2ketosis

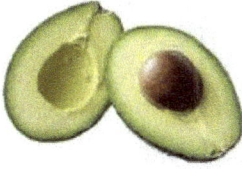

1. Avocado

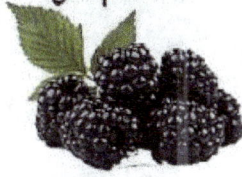

2. Blackberries

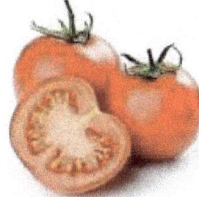

3. Tomatoes

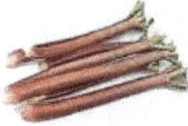

4. Rhubarb

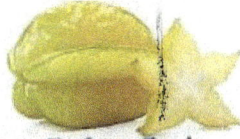

5. Star Fruit

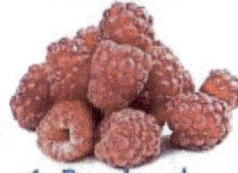

6. Raspberries

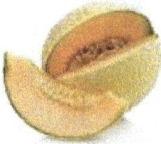

7. Cantaloupe

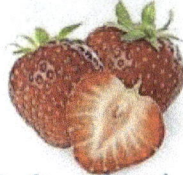

8. Strawberries

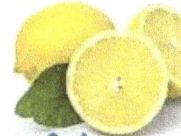

9. Lemon

Ketosis is not harmful, though sometimes people confuse it with the ketoacidosis that a diabetic patient may have. The ketoacidosis results when a diabetic patient's body has excess glucose and uses fat for energy because it has no insulin to process the glucose. I ask all of my clients to watch YouTube or Facebook videos produced by ZDogMD or other wonderful nutritionists to get more information, since it's easier to process important information if it's sugar coated with flashy visuals and humor. I primarily recommend ketogenic diets to my clients during the maintenance phase of weight reduction and usually recommend intermittent fasting alongside it. I've found my clients remain less hungry because they don't get the insulin spikes from carbs. And I usually recommend intermittent fasting alongside the keto diet (more on this below).

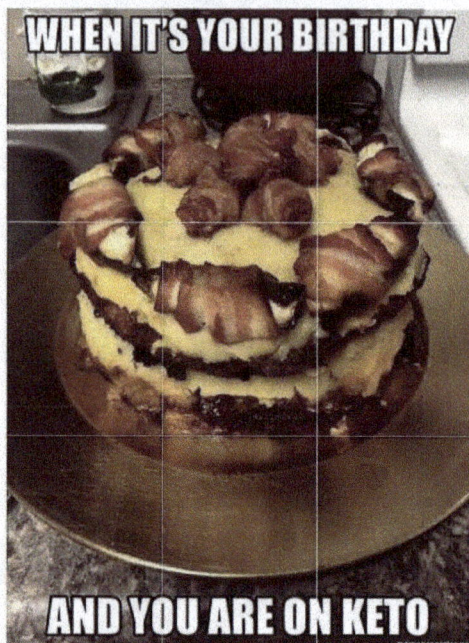

Ketogenic diets have to be undertaken with care and under the supervision of your physician. Some of the most common side effects are increased cholesterol and kidney stones. The way to avoid high levels of cholesterol is to learn to eat polyunsaturated fats from rich food sources like olive oil and avocados. I tell my clients that the magic in all these diets—whether we are talking about Mediterranean, ketogenic, vegan, paleo, etc.—is that they all eliminate refined sugar and ultra-processed food products and replace them with real whole foods. And that is the secret sauce. Since refined sugar is metabolized in the liver like a toxin, high levels of sugar in the diet can lead to insulin resistance and obesity. I believe that the obesity epidemic in America increased after people adopted high-carbohydrate diets and gave up high-fat diets, particularly with the increase in sugary sodas and drinks and the prevalence of ultra-processed foods. Understand that a can of Campbell's soup may have a lot of processed sugars and be bad for you, and a grass-fed steak may be a healthier choice. Fructose is also present in fruit, but it is wrapped in the matrix of the fruit's fiber and, therefore, doesn't cause the sugar high and resultant insulin spike. This is the reason why eating good old-fashioned fruit is better than juicing fad diets, because juicing releases the sugars from the fruit's fiber matrix, leading your body to metabolize it too quickly.

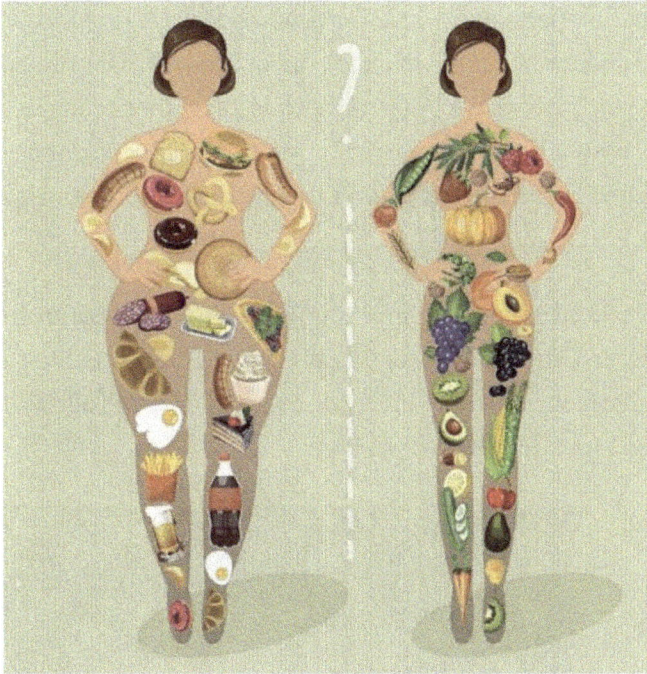

hcgmiami
San Diego, California

···

76 likes

hcgmiami Our HCG Diet Plan will change your body from the inside and out. Visit our site for more information. #Hcgdiet #hcg... more

Calorie Restriction Diets

The name kind of speaks for itself—instead of (or in addition to) changing the type of food that you eat (as ketogenic diets do), this approach reduces your overall caloric intake. If you eat fewer calories than your body burns in a given period, you will lose weight. If it were really that easy, of course, we'd all already be at our ideal weight, and I wouldn't need two CoolSculpting machines in my anti-aging practice. (Two is faster than one!) Sometimes the brain doesn't always cooperate with our weight loss plans and plays tricks on us, like slowing down our metabolism when we reduce our caloric intake and creating intense cravings after the weight has come off. Humans evolved in contexts where food supplies were unreliable, which likely made these features adaptive. However, in our current food environment—where we have access to more calories than we need—these adaptations thwart us more than help us. So the trick is to find a calorie restriction diet that works with your body and brain instead of against them.

I especially recommend the HCG diet, one of the most popular and best-known calorie restriction diets. It's perfectly suited for food addicts. It provides strict caloric restriction and gives a rehabilitated eating schedule to clients who simply can't stop eating junk, unintentionally or otherwise. HCG refers to human chorionic gonadotropin, a hormone measured in women who are pregnant. It floods the body during pregnancy but is present only in trace amounts otherwise. (Don't worry, the HCG calorie restriction diet can also be used in men.)

The diet involves subcutaneously injecting HCG in highly controlled (tiny) doses to calm the appetite centers, and then patients eat only recommended foods—mostly vegetables, meats, fish, and some fruits. The HCG diet should only be followed for three or six weeks at a time, and no more than twice a year.

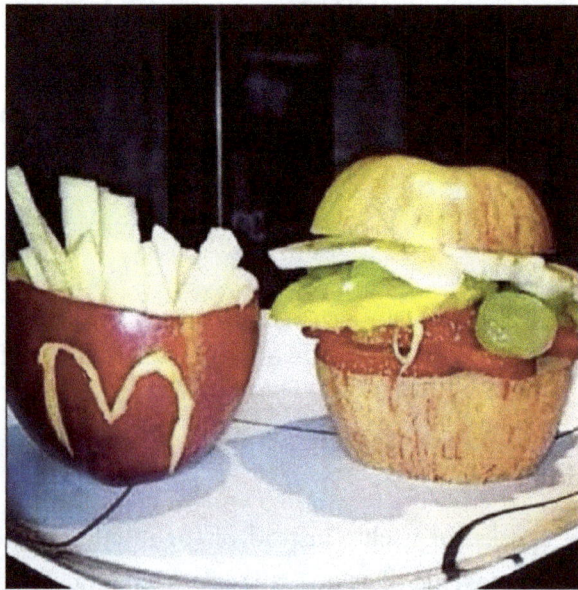

An HCG Happy Meal!

When I administer the HCG diet, I also don't allow any sugars or artificial sweeteners in order to avoid insulin spikes, which can make you hungry. I have prescribed this diet to clients (and used it myself intermittently) over the past eight years. We always monitor clients' blood work prior to starting and during treatment. By following this protocol, I have not encountered any serious side effects. I must have successfully treated over a thousand clients and have almost a 90% satisfaction rate in short-term weight reduction with this approach. I also have a similarly high rate in long-term weight reduction when HCG is combined with other nonsurgical solutions, such as CoolSculpting and a healthy diet. It's one of the best treatments for food addiction clients when coupled with weekly biofeedback in the office.

HCG can cause women to have a heavier menstrual period for the first few days, but this can be controlled simply by not injecting HCG for the first two days of the period. *It's one of the best treatments for food addiction clients, in my opinion, when coupled with weekly biofeedback that we recommend and administer in my office.* The only other bothersome part of HCG is that your body can develop a tolerance to HCG, so after three or four treatments, it often no longer works as well. To maximize the efficacy of the HCG calorie restriction diet, you should also avoid consuming alcohol for the three- to six-week period when the hormone is being injected.

I love to give my clients B12/MIC shots to really boost their energy and metabolism while their bodies are busy fighting their own fat cells and converting them into energy.

And I also strongly recommend concurrent CoolSculpting, a nonsurgical procedure that can eliminate 10% to 15% of your fat cells in treated areas, leading to an overall reduction in fat cells. This is really important because most diets don't eliminate fat cells but only shrink the cell size, so the weight comes back quickly if you start eating carelessly again. CoolSculpting, unlike calorie restriction, kills fat cells by freezing them, and then your body's immune system eliminates the dead fat cells, reducing the likelihood that lost weight will be regained once you come off the calorie restriction diet.

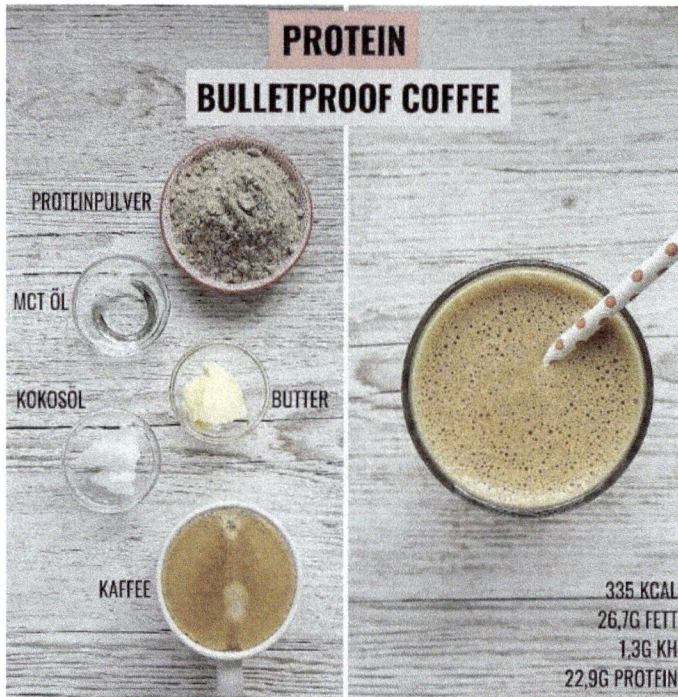

PROTEIN
BULLETPROOF COFFEE

PROTEINPULVER

MCT ÖL

KOKOSÖL   BUTTER

KAFFEE

335 KCAL
26,7G FETT
1,3G KH
22,9G PROTEIN

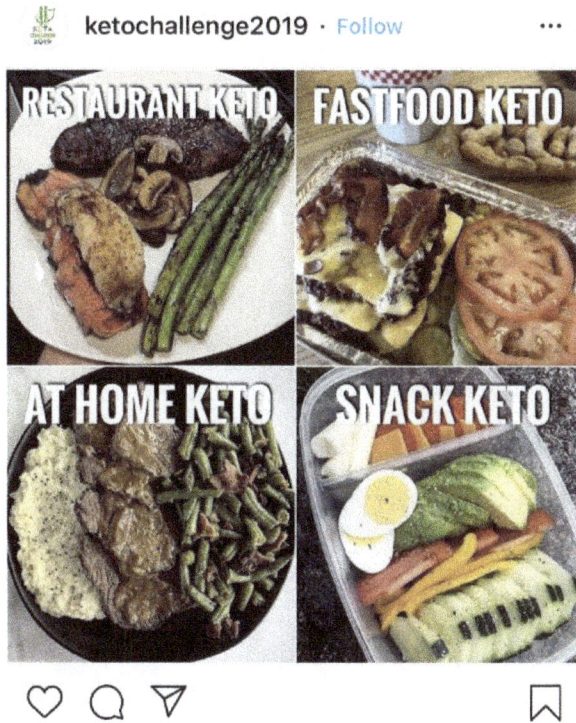

ketochallenge2019 · Follow

1,849 likes

ketochallenge2019 😱 THIS IS HOW EASY KETO IS! DOESN'T GET ANY BETTER THAN THIS... more

Intermittent Fasting

As a child growing up in an Islamic country, I fasted during daylight hours one month each year (the holy month of Ramadan). Everyone fasts except the elderly, the infirm, very young children, and women who are menstruating, pregnant, or breastfeeding. I used to detest these restrictions, but I also enjoyed eating the delicious food we had in the evenings to break the fast. After losing a few pounds initially, our excessive evening eating kept us from losing any more weight.

Fast-forward to a different continent and a different time (2018). I encountered intermittent fasting via Dave Aspery's Bulletproof diet books and talks. I tried it myself since keeping my weight and my clients' weight down was super important for the continued success of my practice. HCG is great and all, but clients kept putting the weight they lost back once going back to their old lifestyles. I would remind them (and myself) that you can never cheat your way out of a bad diet. It's just that simple. So I started prescribing intermittent fasting as part of the weight maintenance part of my HCG and keto diet plans. It helped my clients, and even me, to keep the weight off.

Intermittent fasting is a fancy term for not snacking and more specifically refers to the idea that you should maximize the time between your last meal of the day and your breakfast on the following day. Sometimes it also involves skipping a meal, like breakfast. If you can compress all of your food consumption into eight hours (starting at 11:00 a.m. and finishing by 7:00 p.m., for instance), then you can engage in intermittent fasting. Your body enters a ketogenic state during the fasting period and stabilizes blood sugar levels, thereby helping with progressive weight reduction and maintenance (and increased mental focus—a nice bonus).

FASTING TIPS:

GET YOUR SLEEP

STAY SUPER HYDRATED

GET YOUR ELECTROLYTES IN

GO ON WALKS OR MEDITATE & STAY

OUT OF KITCHEN

Since I started following Dave Aspery, I have integrated this aspect of his dietary philosophy into many people's lifestyles and carefully explain all the details. (I have also made Aspery's Bulletproof coffee an essential part of my morning routine.) With my patients, I routinely examine detailed blood reports and their hormonal and vitamin levels before I advise how to start modifying their lifestyles. There's a dizzying array of relevant information, so it's important to emphasize the importance of working with a medical doctor or nutritionist.

Food is not just calories, it is information. It talks to your DNA and tells it what to do. The most powerful tool to change your health, environment and entire world is your fork.

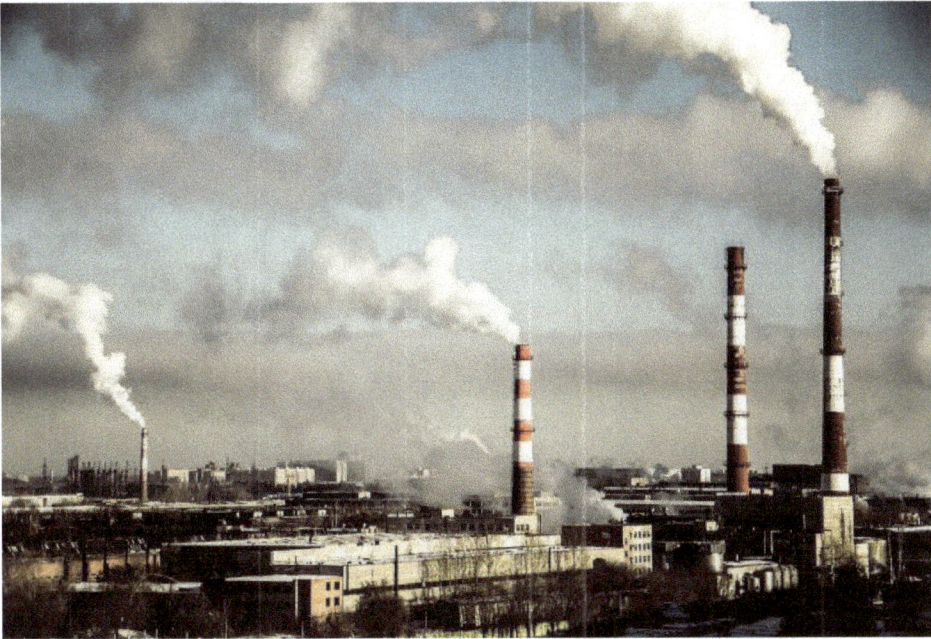

YOU ARE *ALSO* WHAT YOU DRINK AND INHALE

Living in a polluted city, smoking, vaping, and drinking too much alcohol will also affect your weight and your health. Sometimes people don't hear the warning signs or don't take them seriously. The daze of being in the matrix of their existence is simply too intense, and they can't shake it out of their minds. I have personally committed serious errors in my own decision-making, which has led me to consume products that were harmful for my body.

I used to be a smoker, and even though I quit when I became pregnant in 1998, I started again during residency training in 2006, when I was under tremendous stress. I tried quitting a few times (unsuccessfully) and finally quit in 2009, before my daughter could know of my bad habit. I avoided cigs for several years, even through my acrimonious divorce in 2011, but when my ex-husband suddenly died in 2014, I started smoking again. My daughter was 15 at that time and went into a period of severe mourning and grief. While helping my daughter through this, I also managed two separate businesses and felt the stress compounding.

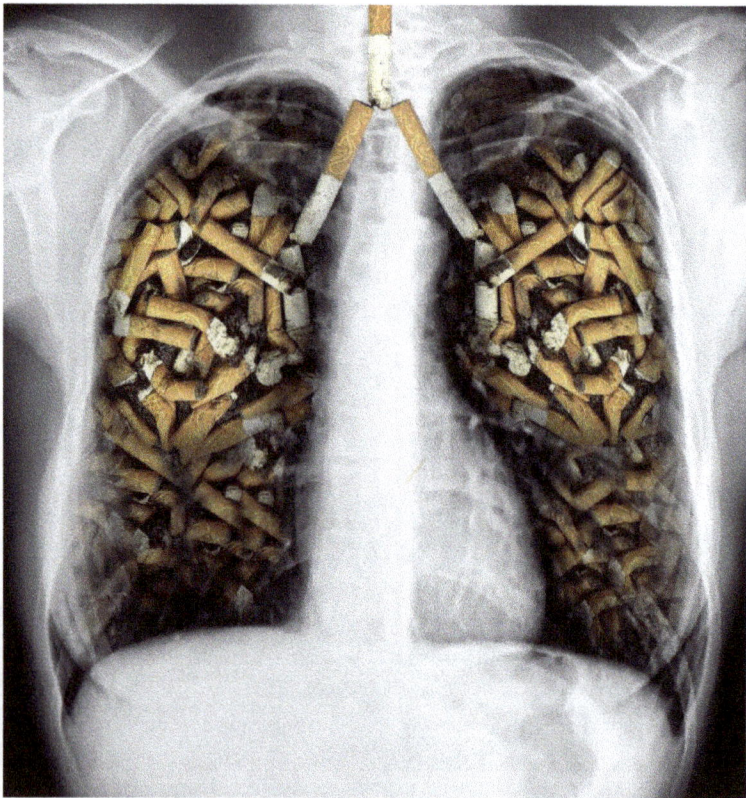

It started innocuously enough: first vaping pens, then hookah. And then I switched back to cigs, and I was hooked again. It took me years to quit again (2018). I tried medications like Contrave and transcranial magnetic stimulation (TMS) therapy to help me kick the habit, but all the while I was worried that I would gain weight if I stopped.

Smoking, alcohol, and food are often used to relieve emotional or mental pain or escape the boredom of routine life and its silly burdens, but at other times as necessary medications to relieve emotional or mental pain.

I wasn't a bored housewife. I was in physical and mental distress from working long shifts in the hospital while raising a daughter in a hostile home.

Smoking and drinking were meant to relieve the stress and mental and emotional exhaustion. Of course, none of this really helped me. And I was acutely aware of the harm that I was causing my body. So I quit smoking in 2018 and stopped drinking alcohol in 2019.

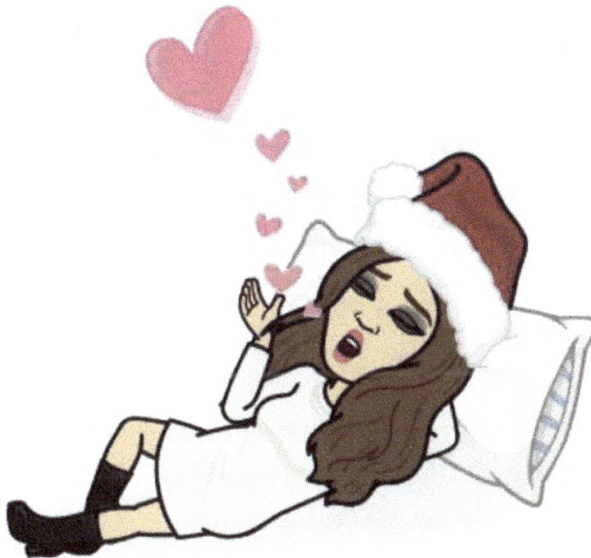

Successfully quitting required me to develop healthier coping mechanisms. *I learned Transcendental Meditation and Vipassana, along with other breathing techniques.*

But during my periods of stress in the past, I hadn't really been regulating my meditation and sleep requirements. I know how important they are, and I allow my body to self-regulate my sleep and wake cycles automatically now. I found a correlation between my own sleep cycles and weight gain and weight loss. This has led me to monitor my own sleep daily and to remind my clients to set aside sleep hours for better health and continued weight maintenance.

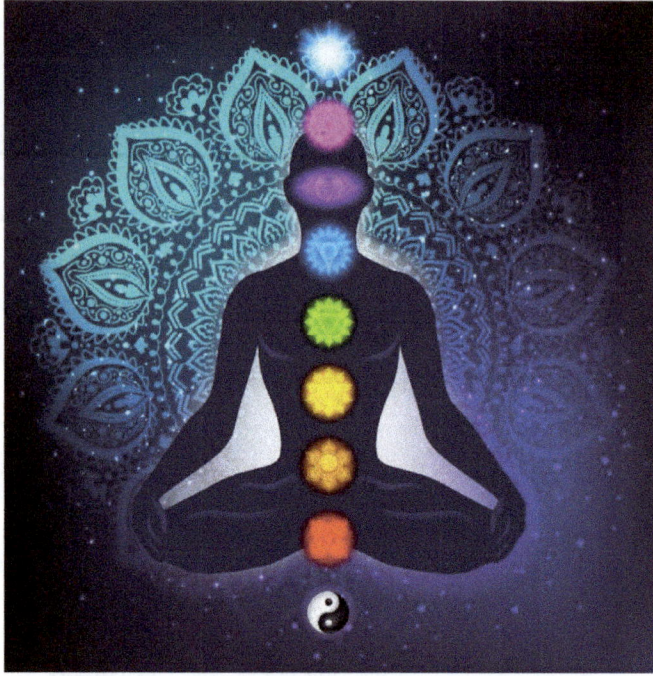

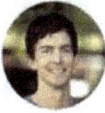

Kurt Rawlins
@KrawlFitness

💥HOW TO LOSE FAT 💥

1985: Don't eat fat

1995: Eat more carbs on workout days

2004: Eat 6x/day

2009: Only eat stuff that was here 10,000 years ago

2015: Skip breakfast

2017: Put butter in your coffee

2019: Eat lots of fat and no carbs

Forever: Calorie deficit

DO YOU AGREE?

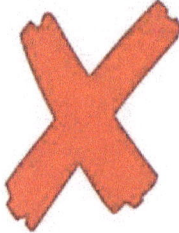

WHAT PEOPLE THINK IS DIFFICULT

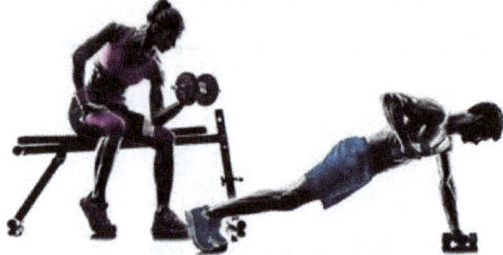

WHAT IS ACTUALLY DIFFICULT

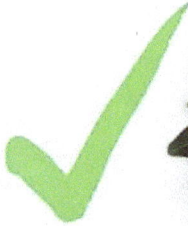

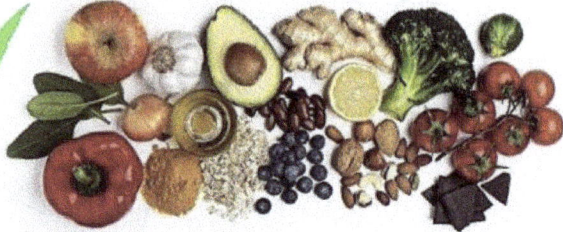

CHAPTER 7

SKIN-TIGHTENING DEVICES

In my experience, most skin-tightening devices are really expensive and either require repeated treatments or are simply ineffective in providing the desired relief a client seeks. *Companies climb over each other to convince you that their product is somehow different and offers unique benefits, but in the face of ground reality, they all fall miserably flat on their faces.*

But, not a lot of options are available yet. Once the skin starts losing its natural elasticity due to aging (because our body stops producing the amount of collagen that it once used to), the skin does start sagging. It is, however, possible to slow down the progression with some devices like Ultherapy or any of the microneedling plus radiofrequency laser combination devices.

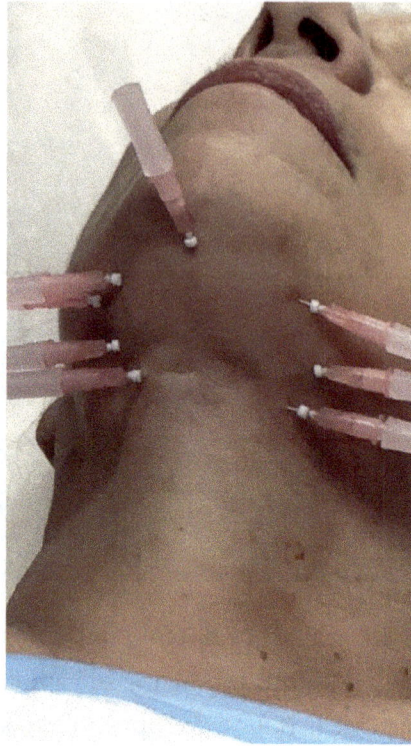

The number of people seeking to prevent sagging hasn't changed much since I started in this industry. In my personal opinion, cosmetic surgery should be avoided until later in life, and only when nothing else works. It's good practice to address body dysmorphia issues so that the patient accepts realistic goals of healthy aging. This prevents most patients from remaining dissatisfied with their results. Sometimes their self-perception might never change, despite costly and painful surgical procedures. This is why I firmly believe that all clients considering surgery should obtain cognitive behavioral therapy before and after the procedures for better long-term wellness.

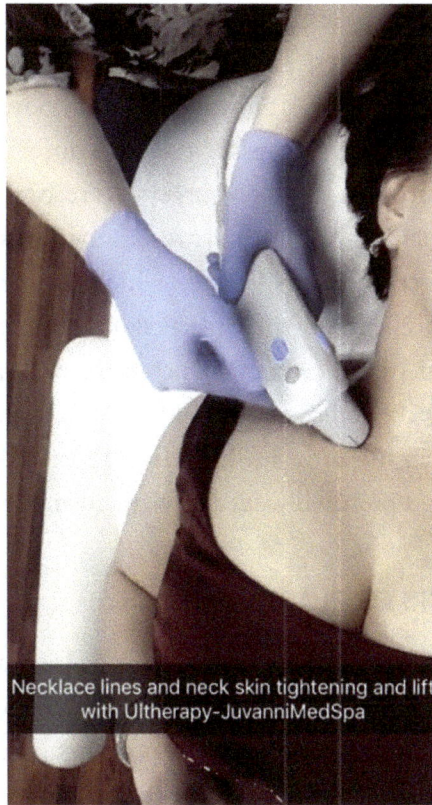

Necklace lines and neck skin tightening and lift with Ultherapy-JuvanniMedSpa

Because having psoriasis made skin such an important part of my life, I've had a long-standing interest in dermatology. As I started my own wellness center, I regularly followed Dr. Doris Day, a true leader in the industry and a voice of sanity in the crazy race for new and better procedures. Her radio shows and books guide countless people to improve the way they age without resorting to surgical solutions unless they become necessary (for example, when the eyelids start drooping, causing vision impairment). I recommend both her books highly. *Forget the Facelift* was one of the first books that led me to develop faith in skincare and skin restoration with nonsurgical procedures, such as fillers and neuromodulators.[39]

WHAT DEVICES ARE AVAILABLE NONSURGICALLY, AND WHAT PROCEDURES WORK IF DONE REGULARLY

Lasers, microneedling devices, and targeted sound waves can be used to tighten and firm up loose skin. I chose to use a variety of skin tightening devices in my practice (e.g.,

---

[39] See Doris Day, *Forget the Facelift: Turn Back the Clock with a Revolutionary Program for Ageless Skin*, (New York: Avery, 2006).

Ulthera, Vivace, PDO threads, etc.). Ultherapy is an ultrasound technology which delivers energy via targeted sound waves, causing micro-injuries to the deeper layers of the skin layer, resulting in skin firmness and tightening as the body repairs the micro-injuries over the next few months. Since it's a nonsurgical procedure, there is minimal to no swelling and tolerable discomfort compared to surgery. I recommend it once or twice a year depending on how much someone can afford, since this treatment is not covered by insurance yet. I also recommend Vivace, which is a microneedling device with a radiofrequency laser, to clients as their facial skin begins to age. It is quickly becoming popular among my patients since they notice improved skin tone and tightening. But neither device promises miraculous or similar results as cosmetic surgery. But with the continued competition in this area, I just remain hopeful that there will be better-quality tightening devices before I personally need or want cosmetic surgery.

THE WHYS AND WHENS OF PLASTIC SURGERY

Research advises us to delay cosmetic surgery for as long as possible. Because more and more humans are living beyond 80 years of age in the United States, and skin elasticity gets much worse when you are older, it's better to keep surgical options open for ourselves when we are much older. I tell my clients to try and prevent surgery till at least 65. Hopefully, noninvasive techniques will get even more sophisticated in the coming years, so surgeries only become necessary for deformities or for overdue anti-aging treatment.

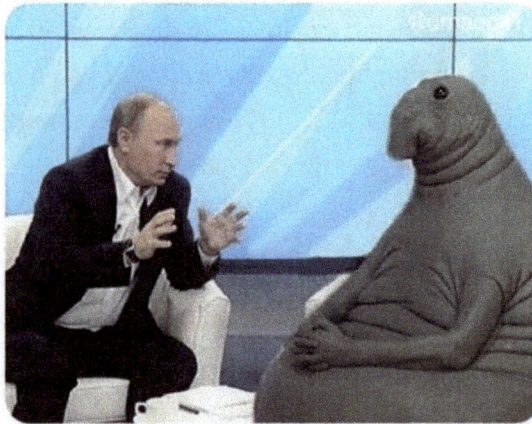

My surgeon trying to explain that a 5th tummy tuck isn't the best option

But why is skin tightening so important? Scientists and biologists are turning to epigenetics to explain and understand aging. It is currently being hypothesized that when people start looking old and their brain perceives them as old, it initiates a cascade of algorithms which sets the body to start manifesting the diseases related to old age. I agree with almost all of these theories. I have followed illustrious neuroscientists like Eric Kandel (who won a Nobel prize for his work).[40] Also, the research and works by David Sinclair and David Eagleman shine light on the capabilities of our magnificent brains and the power that our self-perception carries.

---

[40] See Eric Kandel, *The Age of Insight: The Quest to Understand the Unconscious in Art, Mind, and Brain, from Vienna 1900 to the Present*, (New York: Random House, 2012).

Gift Certificate

Happy Holidays from Juvanni Med Spa!!

This Certificate entitles you to $100 off any service at Juvanni Med Spa with the purchase of the hard cover book & $75 off any service with the purchase of the soft cover book.

To redeem please bring book in with your appointment, please Do Not rip certificate out of book

Certificate expires December 1st, 2020

Sofia Din M.D.

1086 N. Broadway, Suite 80

Yonkers NY, 10701

www.juvanni.com

Call: (914)368-6609

Text: (914)646-2690

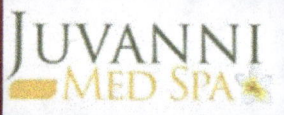

JUVANNI
MED SPA

CHAPTER 8

FIND YOUR MISSING PIECES:
FIND YOUR TRIBE AND UNFOLLOW THE JONESES

The fault, dear Brutus, is not in our stars,
But in ourselves, that we are underlings.

—William Shakespeare, Julius Cesar (I, i, 140–141)

GOING DEEP FOR LIFELONG HEALTH

Throughout this book, I have employed expansive notions of health, both physical and mental; not just avoiding or treating disease, but experiencing full physical functionality, well-being, and vitality throughout a long and productive life; not just avoiding pathology, but being at peace with yourself and motivated by realistic aspirations you set for yourself rather than seeking to live up to goals that are not your own. In paying attention to both physical and mental health, I have also sought to draw attention to the complex interconnections between the two.

For instance, for the sake of physical health and well-being, you should eat real food. Eating well requires, among other things, not engaging in hedonic eating—eating for pleasure instead of the intrinsic contentment derived from eating well-prepared meals that nourish us. Eat because you're hungry, not because you're anxious, craving, bored, or trying to compensate for a lack of contentment.

But avoiding or overcoming hedonic eating may involve identifying and addressing the sources of our cravings or our unhappiness. This may lie in what our diet has done to our bodies and brains. But the sources of our cravings may also stem from a lack of other sources of intrinsic satisfaction in our lives.

To take another example, if you unconsciously internalize an idea of yourself as old and weak, responding with implicit bias against the image that looks back at you from the mirror, your body and behavior may begin to conform to your unconscious self-perception. Maintaining vitality across an extended lifespan requires maintaining an understanding of ourselves as vital, and this may depend on appearing reasonably vital to ourselves and others. The connections go both ways and often move in a self-reinforcing circle: physical health supports psychological health. Mental and physical health are inseparable.

So throughout this book, I advocate for an integrated approach to anti-aging, moving back and forth between an overall philosophy of well-being and healthcare and more specific advice on a variety of anti-aging procedures and strategies including, but certainly not limited to, Botox. This approach aims to foster health, vitality, productivity, and flourishing across a complete and long lifespan. It recommends an innovative approach to medicine, concentrating on preventing disease and maintaining physical functionality, to accompany the lifespan revolution. I have argued that this approach needs to be readily available to all, integrated into 21st century medical education, and covered by insurers. I have also offered advice about how and when to use the various aesthetic procedures I feature in my anti-aging clinic based on the hypothesis that maintaining a flourishing appearance allows us to flourish actually—physically and psychologically—over a complete life.

Finally, I also emphasized a variety of more philosophical, sociological, and psychological claims about taming your body dysmorphia demons before turning to aesthetic procedures, as well as resisting the efforts of the food industrial complex to get us addicted to 'food' products that undermine overall health. Even though culture, industry, and especially social media lead us to internalize unrealistic body and beauty norms at the same time that they tempt us to eat in ways that undermine our health, we must learn to develop realistic self-conceptions and habits, including a realistic understanding of healthy aging. Recognizing the importance of all of this, and acting at the same time on all these fronts, is what I mean, then, by an integrated approach to anti-aging.

In this concluding chapter, I pivot back to the more philosophical vein. The theme here is that leading a long, healthy, productive life requires not only maintaining physical and psychological health but also having deep sources of contentment, meaning, and connection in your life. Having said that, I also want to begin with the necessary caveat that, on these issues, medicine has no particular claim to insight, and medical doctors can lead shallow lives devoid of meaning just as easily as anyone else. As my boyfriend sometimes says, "Dammit, Din! You're a doctor, not a guru!"

(If you're unfamiliar with the "Dammit, Jim" meme from the original Star Trek, you can Google it or see the image below . . .)

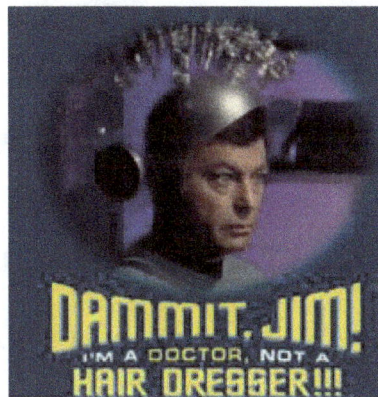

What follows is not based on my certifications, only on experiences in my personal life, what has worked with my patients, and what I've learned from medical research. If finding sources of meaning and fulfillment in life were something that could be easily distilled in a single chapter of a book, there wouldn't be whole self-help sections in bookstores and on Amazon.

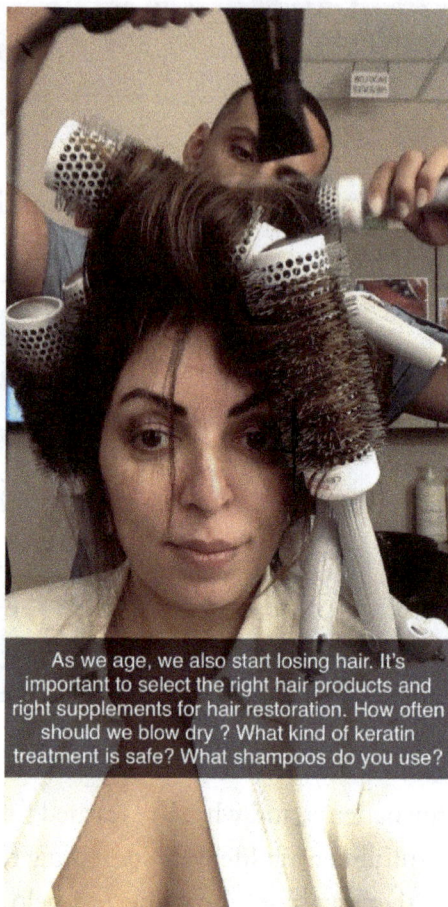

As we age, we also start losing hair. It's important to select the right hair products and right supplements for hair restoration. How often should we blow dry ? What kind of keratin treatment is safe? What shampoos do you use?

Modern science is increasingly revealing to us the importance of emotional health. The frenzy of new information, technology, and the dizzying speed of progress will require us to have significant emotional fortitude and resilience.[41] I have treated hundreds of people with generalized anxiety disorder, and to my dismay, most of the treatments offered to people are medications of limited efficacy. In my clinical experience, my patients with anxiety disorders often benefit more from learning skills like meditation, cognitive behavioral therapy (CBT), and emotional intelligence (EI) workshops that alert them not only to their triggers but the underlying sources of their anxiety. EI workshops are relatively new and not widely available—and the good ones are expensive, since a good workshop follows clients for three to six months. They are currently not covered by most health insurance policies. (One of the workshops in development for Hagar's Foundation

---

[41] These themes are emphasized by Yuval Noah Harari in *21 Lessons for the 21st Century*, especially Part V, (New York: Spiegel & Grow, 2018).

for Single Mothers will help women seeking to get back on their feet and to improve their emotional intelligence.)

I want to encourage you to think carefully about the sources of true satisfaction in your life and the pieces you may be missing. But if you are in a position to also start studying meditation (I especially recommend Transcendental Meditation), seek CBT counseling, or participate in an EI workshop, these options will certainly facilitate your success in identifying and setting down the road to eliminating your missing pieces.

What I can offer here is as much negative as positive, since it focuses in part on what to avoid and how our society often encourages us to focus on superficial markers of success instead of deep sources of fulfillment. But let me start with a simple overview of the positive ideas. To benefit from anti-aging procedures, to eat well, and to be satisfied with your appearance, energy, and vitality—in short, to achieve complete physical and mental health—it is necessary, not only to take care of yourself in the many ways outlined in this book, but also to examine yourself to see if your life is missing sources of deep intrinsic satisfaction.

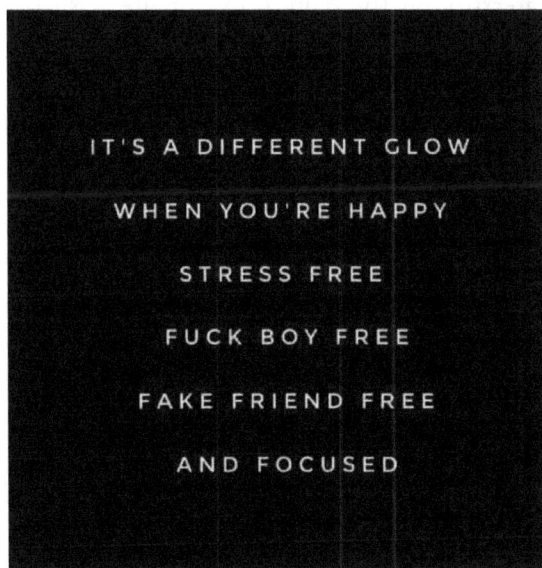

> IT'S A DIFFERENT GLOW
>
> WHEN YOU'RE HAPPY
>
> STRESS FREE
>
> FUCK BOY FREE
>
> FAKE FRIEND FREE
>
> AND FOCUSED

The following is a laundry list of typical sources of intrinsic meaning and satisfaction that can be reviewed in a process of introspective reflection to see where your current contentment comes from and to see which pieces might be missing. Please don't think you can immediately go out and acquire everything you don't already have. But if in your reflection you find that your life does not contain as much intrinsic happiness as it should, and that this is perhaps driving you to seek happiness in unhealthy and unfulfilling ways, then maybe you can begin to explore whether you would be better off investing more time and energy in *some* of these potential sources of intrinsic satisfaction:

1. Forging connections with other people and maintaining regular, meaningful, in-person contact with friends, family, and loved ones.
2. Belonging and contributing to something bigger than yourself.
3. Contributing in ways that help those in need, and displaying generosity when you can.
4. Finding outlets for creativity and self-expression (painting, dancing, cooking, teaching, writing, gardening, fixing up old cars—the possibilities are endless).
5. Setting and pursuing long-term life goals according to your own standards and ideas, not just to meet anyone else's expectations (especially not society's).
6. Engaging in lifelong learning in a field you find exciting or rewarding (from literature, philosophy, and physics to cooking, gardening, and ornithology).
7. Integrating meditation and other relaxation techniques into your daily routine to release toxic stress and figure out what's really going on with you.
8. Getting enough sleep and exercise, and rewarding activity on a daily basis.
9. Regularly interrupting the daily grind of life with a walk in a park, a trip to a museum, a concert, a short vacation, etc.

No doubt, I'm leaving much out here, and clearly not everyone finds lasting satisfaction in the same sources. So be sure to note this final item on the list:

10. Searching and experimenting to find what works to make life meaningful for you.

For much of human history, it wouldn't have been necessary to assemble such a list for people. It's not just that thinking about health, well-being, and contentment are high-class problems, but also that attention to meaning and satisfaction, connection, and commitment to something bigger than yourself was built into the very fabric of many societies and cultures. But modern life tends to prioritize other pursuits, sending us to the wrong places to find happiness.

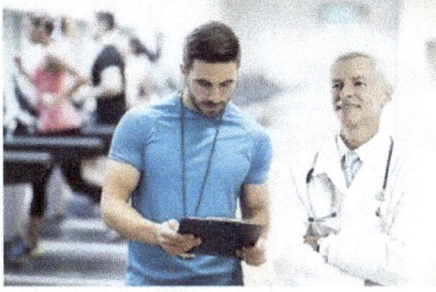

≡ Ⓜ *THE MANSE TIMES* 🔍

Plastic Surgeon Hires Personal Trainer After His Competitor Gets Over 700 Likes On Recent Gym Selfie

Written By Dr Na'omi | *Contact*

♥ ○ ◁   🔖

Liked by **botoxbunny** and **317 others**

WHAT MONEY CAN'T BUY

Every year the U.N. publishes the World Happiness Report, which ranks the countries of the world according to their relative happiness. *If you look at one of these reports, you may be surprised to find that the richest countries are not the happiest. In fact, there is no correlation between wealth and happiness among the richer countries of the world.*[42]

Fascinating research by two epidemiologists and public health doctors in Britain, Richard Wilkinson and Kate Pickett, shows that past a certain threshold ($20,000 per person per year), there is no relationship between wealth and happiness. Whereas the authors of the U.N. report focus on a variety of factors (including community and prosocial behavior on the positive side, and social media use and addiction on the negative side), Pickett and Wilkinson hone in on a single variable: the degree of relative inequality in a state or country. More wealth does not make a society healthier, but greater inequality makes its residents less healthy, both physically and psychologically.

These are odd and controversial findings. What's going on here? Wilkinson and Pickett's work gains support from the emerging field of inequality studies, and the overall evidence

---

[42] See World Happiness Report 2019, Ch.2, figure 2.7, (https://worldhappiness.report/ed/2019/changing-world-happiness/).

accumulated is extremely persuasive. It is also important for each of us as we think through what kind of society we want to have (for instance, more or less rich, or more or less equal) and what ends we should pursue to flourish across all the stages of life (for instance, more wealth or greater community).[43]

Among the findings emphasized in this literature is that different societies have different degrees of relative social distance between their members (i.e., how many common experiences, problems, and contexts people share). This social distance affects the level of cooperation, trust, and reciprocity among people. After all, it's much easier to sympathize and cooperate with others, especially strangers, if you assume that you all have a fair bit in common. The more equal the society, the less social distance, meaning members experience more trust and reciprocity and have a greater sense of social belonging and solidarity—keys to health and happiness.[44] Alternatively, the more unequal a society, the more its members tend to mistrust and compete with each other, which undermines the happiness for both the losers and the winners racing for social success.

Another factor concerns social evaluative threat, a kind of status anxiety that is experienced when you worry that people are looking down on you based on makers of social status, such as the kind of clothes you're wearing, or car you drive, the phone you're on, or the color of your skin.[45] In more unequal societies, relative status matters more, and so people are more frequently subject to this kind of social evaluation and the stress it generates. This stress triggers cortisol production, which in turn affects both brain and body chemistry in highly deleterious ways. In this way, high levels of inequality lead to population-wide decreases in both mental and physical health, in both the rich and the poor and everyone in between. The result is not only a less happy but also a less healthy society, which is why Pickett and Wilkinson treat inequality not primarily as an issue of social justice so much as one of public health.

Finally, and perhaps most destructively, unequal societies produce higher levels of downward prejudice—that is to say, people looking down at others in order to feel better about themselves. This is sometimes referred to as social bicycling because you push

[43] See Kate Pickett and Richard Wilkinson, *The Spirit Level: Why Equality is Better for Everyone*, (New York: Penguin, 2010) and *The Inner Level: How More Equal Societies Reduce Stress, Restore Sanity and Improve Everyone's Well-Being*, (New York: Penguin, 2018).
[44] See, for instance, Robert Putnam, *Our Kids: The American Dream in Crisis*, (New York: Simon Schuster, 2015).
[45] See especially Claude Steele, *Whistling Vivaldi: How Stereotypes Affect Us and What We Can Do*, (New York: WW Norton, 2010).

down—not on pedals but on others—in order to get ahead. The result, Wilkinson and Pickett postulate, is that more unequal societies experience higher levels of insecure self-esteem. *If one of the main reasons you feel good about yourself is because you believe you are superior to others on some fairly superficial measure of social status, your sense of self is not built on solid ground.*

We all have a basic human need to love and respect ourselves, and because we depend on others to confirm our self-conceptions, sources of self-regard vary from individual to individual and according to what one's society deems is worthy of respect.[46]

A more unequal society, perhaps unwittingly, encourages us to hang our sense of self-worth on attributes that are superficial, not intrinsically satisfying, and often quite unstable. As David Bowie put it in his most bitingly bitter song: "What you need you have to borrow." (Fame)

Why the long detour into inequality studies in a chapter on the significance of having intrinsic meaning and contentment in your life and personal well-being for overall, lifelong health? Because almost all of us (except the lucky ones who live in the happiest countries on the planet) are living in societies that are much more unequal than they were 50 years ago, and we are all suffering the consequences.

If your life is missing pieces essential to your overall fulfillment, and you're tempted to turn to money or food or Botox to compensate for what's lacking, you need a better understanding of what will bring you true meaning and fulfillment more than you need more stuff. Social media amplifies and exacerbates the negative effects of more unequal societies, as we increasingly inhabit a digital panopticon, where we feel that we are constantly on display, constantly scrutinized and judged based on the superficial status markers unequal societies encourage us to overvalue.

LOOKING BEYOND MONEY AND WHAT IT BUYS

One of the most insightful descriptions of the perversity of seeking lasting satisfaction through the consumption and display of material goods comes from the great French philosopher Jean Jacques Rousseau when he imagines the history of humankind's

---

[46] I take the phrase from Toni Morrison's *The Source of Self-Regard* (New York: Alfred A. Knopf, 2019). These themes are explored brilliantly by Frederick Neuhouser in *Rousseau's Theodicy of Self-Love: Evil, Rationality, and the Drive for Recognition,* (Oxford: Oxford University Press, 2010).

emergence from the state of nature. Rousseau postulates that we begin to become civilized when we are thrown together in larger communities with a division of labor that makes greater productivity possible. This is how he describes the consequences of the newly emerging wealth:

> In this new state . . . since men enjoyed very great leisure, they used it to procure many new kinds of commodities unknown to their fathers; and that was the first yoke they imposed on themselves without thinking about it, and the first source of the evils they prepared for their descendants. For, besides their continuing thus to soften body and mind, as these commodities had lost almost all their pleasantness through habit, and as they had at the same time degenerated into true needs, being deprived of them became much more cruel than possessing them was sweet; and people were unhappy to lose them without being happy to possess them.[47]

Rousseau's fable illuminates why it is that *seeking satisfaction from commodities—whether it is a new car or phone, an HD TV or clothes—is looking in the wrong place. There is doubtless a thrill in acquiring them and novelty while they are new. But soon we become accustomed to them, and once we do, the thrill tends to fade and is replaced by a craving for another shot of consumption-fueled titillation or outright dependency on the commodity.*

While the language here is perhaps philosophical, the thinking is really quite common sense. Benjamin Franklin, a contemporary of Rousseau's and a man who practically transformed saving money into a religion, said, "A penny saved is a penny earned." But he also advised, "Money has never made man happy, nor will it; there is nothing in its nature to produce happiness. The more of it one has, the more one wants."

---

[47] Jean Jacques Rousseau, *The First and Second Discourses*, Roger Masters, ed., (New York: St. Martins, 1969), p.147.

NOT MY JOB	MY JOB
FIX OR SAVE PEOPLE	LOVE PEOPLE
BE LIKED	BE AUTHENTIC
DO IT ALL	TAKE THE NEXT STEP
PLEASE EVERYONE	SPEAK MY TRUTH
HOLD IT TOGETHER	BREATHE

Modern medical science has perhaps not added much philosophical depth to this discussion, but it has added some understanding of the ways in which the different kinds of rewards associated with different kinds of activities are rooted in the brain and different limbic system pathways. Without getting to wonky here, *I would point out that Robert Lustig, a neuroscientist and endocrinologist, argues that it is essential to differentiate the reward from the contentment pathway. The former relies primarily on the neurotransmitter dopamine, while the latter relies on serotonin.*

Lustig's account explains at a neurobiological level Rousseau's observation about how new commodities produce short-term excitement but not long-term contentment. Dopamine tends to down-regulate its receptors (this accounts for the increased tolerance for stimulants and drugs over time), so that the rush produced on this pathway tends to be short lived and leave one craving for more.[48] But he also points out that many contemporary industries appreciate that fleeting pleasures followed by renewed longing enables a perfect strategy for profits, since consumers keep coming back for more. This is the secret behind the amazing success of the fast and processed food industries, as well as many cell phones, apps, and social media. In short, the fabric of so much of our material life relies on this drive for pleasure, not contentment.

Pulling these themes together, I believe we find a powerful explanation for why, despite our tremendous wealth and the advances in medicine that allow us to live so much longer, we appear not to be getting happier. On the contrary, so many of us report being less satisfied and increasingly anxious, stressed, and lonely. Our country has a growing dependency on antidepressants (a family of medicines of limited efficacy), is ravaged by an opioid crisis, has worrisome suicide rates, and declining life expectancies.[49] All told, it appears that our society strongly encourages us to seek satisfaction from the wrong sources, to compare ourselves with others on the basis of superficial markers of social standing and status, to acquire still more commodities to compensate for the lack of intrinsic satisfaction these pursuits generate, and to work harder and harder to earn the money necessary to keep up with the Joneses on the treadmill of compensatory consumption.[50] It may be time to unfollow the Joneses and find a way to unplug.

---

[48] Lustig, *The Hacking of the American Mind*, op. cit.

[49] See Anne Case and Angus Deaton, "Rising midlife morbidity and mortality, US whites," *Proceedings of the National Academy of Sciences,* Dec 2015, 112 (49) 15078-15083; DOI:.1073/pnas.1518393112.

[50] There are so many good books diagnosing these problems. I'm especially influenced by: Thomas Frank, *Luxury Fever: Why Money Fails to Satisfy in an Era of Excess,* Juliet B. Schor, *The Overspent American: Why We Want What We Don't Need;* and John de Graaf, et. al., *Affluenza: The All-Consuming Epidemic.*

You Unplugged

To look more closely at how society may be misdirecting us, let's look at a single simple but central example: the explosive growth in global social media use over the last decade. According to recent studies, Americans spend upward of 10 hours a day staring at their screens.[51] Let's say that you're not a social media hermit, and you, too, spend some portion of your day checking in on Facebook, Instagram, Twitter, and other social media platforms. I recommend that you ask yourself the following questions:

• How much time am I spending on social media and the internet?
• Is it giving me brief pleasure but ultimately not much lasting happiness, and do I end up longing for more?
• What else could I be doing with my time?
• If I were doing something else with my time, would I be more content at the end of the day?

Recent research suggests that social media and handheld computers (mobile phones), are making us lonelier, less empathetic, more isolated, and less happy—precisely what results from occasional rewards and longing for something deeper.

Sherry Turkle's landmark *Alone Together* and Siva Vaidhyanathan's more recent *Antisocial Media* are among the recent studies that illuminate the sources of discontent in social media.[52] Neither suggest that social media is wholly destructive, and it is worth noting that Turkle, one of the most influential anthropologists of new technology, began her career as a new technology enthusiast. However, both suggest that most users do not get genuine social connections from social media and that real, meaningful communities, friendships, and discussions are being displaced by activities that appear to offer high-tech alternatives but actually lack the essential aspects of real human connection that make them meaningful. The costs of excessive technology use, especially of social media, noted in these studies, are many, and I cannot do justice to all of them her. But a few strike me as particularly relevant to our discussion.

---

[51] See Quentin Fottrell, "People spend most of their waking hours staring at screens," *Market Watch,* August 4, 2018 (https://www.marketwatch.com/story/people-are-spending-most-of-their-waking-hours-staring-at-screens-2018-08-01), (site visited 9/14/2019); and Herring, Mark Y, Social Media and the Good Life: Do They Connect, 2015.

[52] Sherry Turkle, *Alone Together: Why We Expect More from Technology and Less from Each Other,* (New York: Basic Books, 2012); and Siva Vaidhyanathan, *Antisocial Media: How Facebook Disconnects Us and Undermines Democracy,* (Oxford: Oxford University Press, 2018).

Solitude can be understood as time spent alone with yourself to get in touch with how you're doing, what you're feeling, what needs you have that you may not be paying enough attention to, and what sources of joy you may want to be grateful for and cultivate. Solitude is central to emotional development, psychological well-being, and creativity. However, many social media users report being very rarely unplugged from digital connections when alone, making it harder for them to derive benefits from solitude. Instead of practicing self-reflection, they find it hard to resist the temptation to check various apps on their phones.

The constant pull of technology is, as they say, a feature and not a bug. Silicon Valley hires programmers and software designers, but also a small army of psychologists to figure out how to keep you hooked to their devices and the apps they run. For many of us, myself included, the result of social media addiction can be, on the one hand, the substitution of digital social connection for the real thing, and on the other, the loss of enough quality time with yourself to identify the source of your discontent and how to address it. Here, as elsewhere, powerful and largely unregulated industries stack the deck against us, and many children get hooked before they have the mental sophistication or capacities required to resist. It is up to us to think carefully and develop the will, resources, support, and patience necessary to forcefully redirect our attention away from where these attention merchants want to keep it.[53]

Why is social media connectivity such a poor substitute for real human interaction, even with strangers, let alone for the frankly often complicated and sometimes difficult connections we forge and maintain with friends, family, and loved ones? A full answer involves nothing less than a complete understanding of what makes interpersonal relationships one of the deepest sources of lasting human fulfillment, a topic that's been explored in philosophy, psychology, literature, and art for over 2,500 years! However, the migration of direct face-to-face interaction to social media and the greater curation of self-presentation to others it allows is a central fact of modern society. And focusing on this fact alone can help us begin to understand at least some of what makes real, in person relationships such a valuable source of human fulfillment.

Face-to-face interaction allows you to see, well, the face of the person you're interacting with, as well as the way they hold or comport their body. As it turns out, a fair bit of emotional communication is embodied in our facial expressions and other nonverbal cues that convey what we are feeling about what someone else is saying, doing, etc. This reflects deep learning that occurred throughout the development of the human species and our primate ancestors. Strip this away by reducing the other person to a little face on a little screen, and much of the basis for empathy and understanding is lost. Our emotional intelligence proves inadequate, and the relationship shrivels.

When you relate to another in person and directly, typically you give that person your full attention. When you're on one (or more) of your various devices, there's a strong tendency to multitask, which is really just the act of trying to pay partial attention to several activities at once.[54] "Huh? What did you say? Oh yeah . . . sorry . . ." Sound familiar? Part of what makes real, sustained human interaction an irreplaceable source of meaning, love, and growth is precisely the ongoing negotiation of difference within the relationship.

---

[53] See Tim Wu, *The Attention Merchants: The Epic Scramble to Get Inside Our Heads,* (New York: Knopf, 2016).

[54] These themes are developed wonderfully in Nicholas Carr's *The Shallows: What the Internet is Doing to Our Brains,* (New York: W.W. Northon, 2011).

LAUGH LIKE YOU'RE 10
PARTY LIKE YOU'RE 20
TRAVEL LIKE YOU'RE 30
THINK LIKE YOU'RE 40
ADVISE LIKE YOU'RE 50
CARE LIKE YOU'RE 60
LOVE LIKE YOU'RE 70

Being a friend differs from friending someone on social media precisely because it involves the hard work of getting to know a person and revealing yourself to him or her. From that, there's a growth in character and understanding that occurs for both of you. This is what philosophers sometimes refer to as a struggle for recognition. When we get together with old friends, part of the joy in reliving old experiences is not just the sentimental recollection of a particularly fun experience but also revisiting a moment in which together you helped each other discover who you are now. When we substitute online for in-person interaction, and combine it with the absence of solitude being constantly tethered to our phones produces, the result is a loss of emotional range and intimacy.

Finally, there's the spontaneity of in-person interactions—a freedom and fluidity that is often lacking from the presentation of the self to others when mediated by technology. Because true interpersonal connection involves working out the self in relation to someone different from us, it potentially draws creativity—self-creation—out of us. If you have been in an intense conversation with a friend or loved one and been surprised by what's coming out of your mouth, had tears well up in your eyes, or feel a smile on your face even before you fully realize what made you happy, you've experienced the spontaneity and freedom of true interpersonal relations.

For this kind of interpersonal exploration to occur, the context has to allow for spontaneous interaction, and the relationship itself has to sustain the necessary trust.[55] The online presentation of self to others typically lacks the relevant spontaneity, freedom, dialogue, and trust. Instead of enabling the flowing give and take of conversation with someone we know well or want to get to know better, our time online involves selecting and curating the images, the witty remarks, and the memes we want the world to see as a representation of just how smart, cool, clever, or beautiful we are. This can be exhilarating and fun, as well as exhausting and treacherous.

But curating the online self is no substitute for developing yourself through sustained interpersonal connection with others. Nevertheless, many of us now spend more time posting and tweeting and filtering selfies and finding just the right meme than truly spending time with others.

We may have lots of likes and followers and a gleaming online presence, but at the end of the day, we remain lonely, less self-aware and empathetic, and longing for something social media cannot deliver. It's time to look elsewhere for what we are missing.

UNFOLLOWING THE JONESES AND FINDING YOUR OWN SOURCES OF MEANING AND SATISFACTION

I've offered this long detour into philosophy, psychology, and sociology at the end of a book on anti-aging medicine to assist you in diagnosing whether you have missing pieces and, if so, why. I certainly did. Having moved to the U.S. as a young woman to enter an arranged marriage, I quickly realized that my home life was not going to make me happy. So I threw myself into work and eventually had professional and material success. I am eternally grateful for this since it allowed me to attain the independence necessary to escape a destructive relationship, to stand on my own, and to provide the security and stability both my daughter and I needed. But because my marriage was so unhappy—and also probably because I was socialized to believe that current success was only to be valued as a stepping stone to greater success—I became quite compulsive about work, spending all my time and energy in pursuit of growing my practices. It didn't help that I spent a lot of time promoting my practices—and myself—on social media.

---

[55] These themes are developed in profound and original ways by Hannah Arendt in *The Human Condition,* (University of Chicago Press; Enlarged edition, 2018).

Success was sweet in certain respects. I had a big, beautiful house in an affluent suburb with very good schools. I'd driven (and crashed) a succession of Mercedes. I had more clothes in my closets than I could keep track of. But was I happy? Over the last few years, I've come to realize that, while I provided for my daughter, I spent too little time with her in her formative years and outsourced too much of her parenting to others. I experienced great professional success, but did I know what love was? My practices were thriving, I was—and still am—good at what I do, and I get satisfaction out of doing it well. But was I contributing as much as I could to my society and those around me, especially the most vulnerable among us? Was I truly satisfied? I was drinking and eating too much, partying and spending a lot of time on social media, and finding myself still longing for something more fulfilling at the end of the day.

This book is a product of the soul searching I've done to answer these questions over the last few years and the changes I've made in my life as a result. I now drive a Ford, I've made a vow not to shop for new clothes for this entire year, I have rearranged my work schedule to allow more time for myself, and I'm writing, gardening, and feeding the birds that now flock to my backyard. I started dancing and painting, and I plan to also learn cooking. (I want to specialize in healthy 15-minute meals that I can share with working mothers.) I've fallen in love, and my partner and I are building a life together. And I'm trying to make myself more available to my daughter and, often to her chagrin, involving myself more in her life to make up for lost time.

I've also founded a nonprofit foundation, Hagar's Foundation for Single Mothers, and (as I hope you know by now) the proceeds from the book you're about to finish will fund workshops and training for single mothers. Using the skills I've acquired, the knowledge I've accumulated, and the success I've had, I aim to be a resource for other single mothers, which I'm convinced is a worthy life goal for me. It's still a bit scary setting down this new path in the middle of my life, and it certainly isn't the typical immigrant's path. (My accountant, a fellow Desi immigrant, practically bit my head off when I told him I was going to concentrate on not-for-profit work precisely at the moment my businesses were really taking off!) But I'm satisfied at the end of the day, I go to sleep early and sleep well, and I wake up with a sense of mission and purpose.

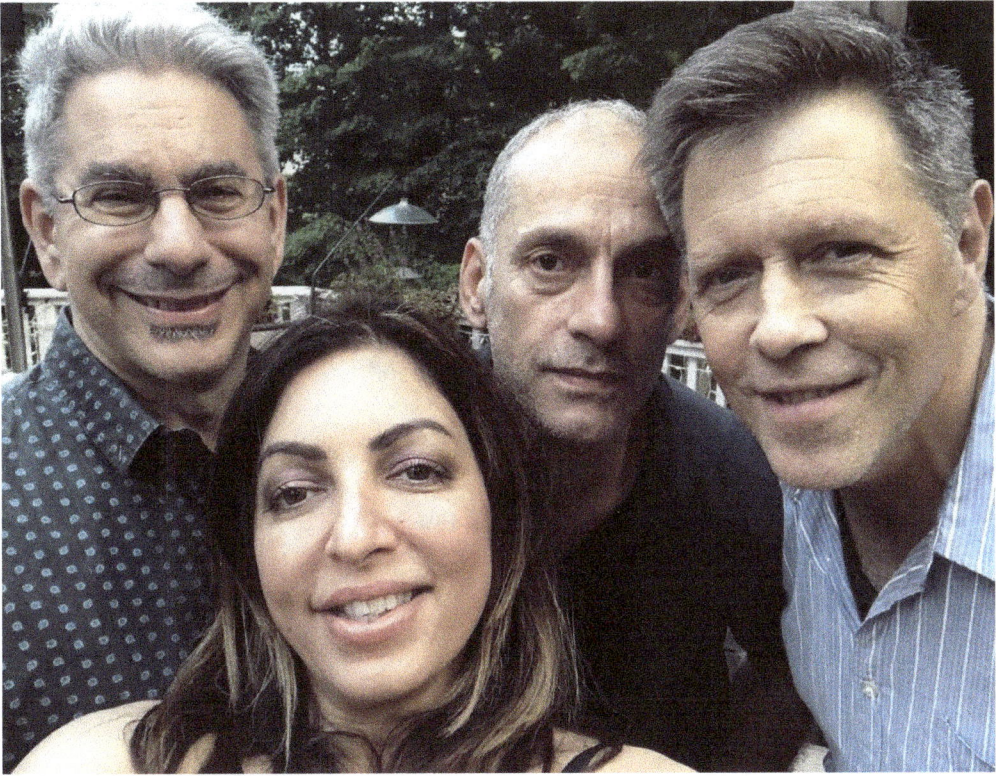

Me with three of Hagar's Foundation's board members and directors, whom we lovingly refer to as Hagar's Angels

Of course, not everyone is in a position to start a charitable foundation, nor would everyone find satisfaction in it even if they were. But I am convinced we are all in a position to assist one another, especially those experiencing vulnerability or suffering, and the kindness we show others not only makes us better, happier people but also contributes to the chain of kindness that radiates out from each act of justice, decency, or charity.

I have also changed my friendship circle in recent years—something made easier by the fact that many of my American friends were originally my ex-husband's friends. Science tells us that good relationships and soul-satisfying friendships will enhance and add years to our lives. This is not new information either. Years of research and tons of money have been spent to come to the advice that my mom (and many others) offer in one sentence: "Follow your heart." (Even though my mom is almost blind, her intuition is razor sharp.)

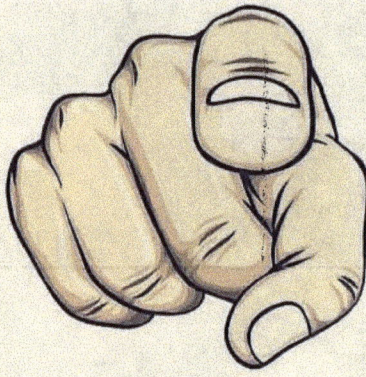

Hey You..

**Stop getting sad over small things
stop getting emotional over
things you can't control
It's time for you to be happy again
You deserve happiness**

A key component of being content is having the feeling of support and belonging, but if you don't identify with the group that you are with now, you might need to find people you better connect with mentally and emotionally. So before you look for your tribe, you must become self-aware. How can you find your tribe if you don't know yourself and you don't know how to connect with others? It certainly wasn't easy for me to build a new circle of friends in the middle of my life and as my career was really heating up. But it has been immensely rewarding, as I am now surrounded by warm people who accept, challenge, encourage, and support me.

My concluding advice to you is this. If you want to lead a long life that is filled with vitality, energy, productivity, and health, examine the life you're leading now and identify the sources of lasting satisfaction, meaning, and happiness in your life. Then project yourself into the closing chapter of your life and pretend to look back on your life. Will this future you feel it was worthwhile that you spent time and energy on those satisfying endeavors more than others? Just as in approaching the food on your plate, take an x-ray of your life to see if what you're consuming and doing is nurturing you. (Do you know where everything you're eating comes from, why you're eating it, and what it's doing for or to you?) I suggest a similar approach in x-raying your life to determine whether its main activities are nurturing your soul or if something is missing. When doing this life x-ray, consider the following questions:

1. How is your self-esteem?
2. Do you feel self-confident?
3. Is love missing in your life?
4. Are the main activities in your life providing you with stable, lasting fulfillment or leaving you longing for more?
5. Are you connected with other people? Are the people you're connected with the right people to help you develop and thrive?
6. Is your life missing its meaning or purpose? Why or why not?
7. Can any missing pieces be found?
8. Is peace of mind missing in your life?

Nothing can trouble us more, except our own imagination or lack of it.

Asking questions like these will set you on the path to greater self-awareness, which is a key component in anti-aging and aging well. Becoming aware of who you are, what you like or dislike, and what you want in life are important aspects of a well-lived life.

If you find yourself motivated by longings and cravings, if you're looking to social media, food, booze, drugs, money, commodities, or Botox for satisfaction and you find yourself still wanting more, maybe you're not tapping the right sources for lasting contentment. While new medical breakthroughs and procedures can help you live longer and maintain vitality across that long life, the age-old lesson that a good life is a life well lived remains as relevant today as ever.

(To be continued)

Index

A

Allergan, 3, 52, 55, 57, 84, 85, 89
Anti-aging, 23, 68

B

Bariatric surgery, 123
Belviq, 121, 122
Body Dysmorphia, 3, 36, 40, 41, 47
Botox, 3, 20, 28, 35, 42, 46, 47, 48, 49, 52, 53, 54, 55, 56, 57, 61, 62, 63, 64, 65, 66, 71, 85, 86, 87, 88, 89, 145, 151, 163
Botulinum Toxin, 56
Brain, 45, 113, 142

C

Contraindications, 54
Contrave, 121, 122, 135
CoolSculpting, 85, 89, 96, 123, 129, 130, 131
CoolSculpting by Zeltiq, 85

D

Dermal Fillers, 74
Desi, 11, 160
Diets, 115, 126, 129
Diplopia (double vision), 54
Dopamine, 153
Dysport, 57, 88

E

Edible Schoolyard, 112
Education, 101, 112
Exercise, 118

F

Face-to-face interaction, 157
Filters, 3, 41, 71
Flourishing, 57

Food, 3, 4, 57, 90, 96, 98, 99, 101, 102, 105, 106, 107, 109, 111, 112, 115
Forget the Facelift, 140
Friendship, 35

G

Group 1, 102, 103, 105, 110
Group 2, 102, 103, 105
Group 3, 103, 105
Group 4, 103, 105

H

Happiness, 112, 149
Health, 47, 78, 111, 144
Hedonic eating, 112
Hierarchy of Needs, 18

I

Implicit, 59
Instagram, 23, 41, 71, 154
Intermittent fasting, 133

J

Jeuveau, 57, 88
Juvanni Med Spa and Anti-Aging Center, 14

K

Ketogenic, 126, 128

M

Medical School, 95
Medicine, 17, 19, 37, 40, 58, 122
Meditation, 136, 147

N

NOVA food classification system, 102
Nutrition, 100, 101, 102, 105, 110

O

Organic, 109, 110

P

Pakistan, 9, 10, 11, 37, 67, 96
Paxil, 28
Phantoms in the Brain, 43
Philosophy, 16, 57
Philosophy of, 57
Physical, 112
Pills, 121

Q

Qsymia, 121, 122

R

Revance, 88

S

Self, 59, 118
Single Mothers, 1, 14, 31, 147, 160
Skillful, 35
Skin, 28, 37, 74, 140
Skin-Tightening Devices, 3, 139
Slow Food, 112
Snapchat, 41, 71
Social Media, 41, 154
Solitude, 155
Substances commonly used in, 72

T

Thinking, 35, 46
True Mirror, 45

U

Ultherapy, 139, 141

V

VB6, 111
Vipassana, 136
Vivace, 141

W

Wellbutrin, 28
Wellness and, 61

X

Xeomin, 57, 88
X-ray Your Plate, 116